Supporting transitions in the early years

Supporting early learning

Series Editors: Vicky Hurst and Jenefer Joseph

The focus of this series is on improving the effectiveness of early education. Policy developments come and go, and difficult decisions are often forced on those with responsibility for young children's well-being. This series aims to help with these decisions by showing how developmental approaches to early education provide a sound and positive basis for learning.

Each book recognizes that children from birth to 6 years old have particular developmental needs. This applies just as much to the acquisition of subject knowledge, skills and understanding as to other educational goals such as social skills, attitudes and dispositions. The importance of providing a learning environment that is carefully planned to stimulate children's own active learning is also stressed.

Through the series, readers are encouraged to reflect on the education being offered to young children, through revisiting developmental principles and using them to analyse their observations of children. In this way, readers can evaluate ideas about the most effective ways of educating young children and develop strategies for approaching their practice in ways that offer every child a more appropriate education.

Published and forthcoming titles:

Liz Brooker: *Supporting Transitions in the Early Years*
Jonathan Doherty and Richard Bailey: *Supporting Physical Development and Physical Education in the Early Years*
Bernadette Duffy: *Supporting Children and Imagination in the Early Years 2nd edition*
Lesley Hendy and Lucy Toon: *Supporting Drama and Role Play in the Early Years*
Vicky Hurst and Jenefer Joseph: *Supporting Early Learning – The Way Forward*
Caroline Jones: *Supporting Inclusion in the Early Years*
Linda Pound and Chris Harrison: *Supporting Music in the Early Years*
Linda Pound: *Supporting Mathematical Development in the Early Years 2nd edition*
Iram Siraj-Blatchford and Priscilla Clarke: *Supporting Identity, Diversity and Language in the Early Years*
John Siraj-Blatchford and Iain MacLeod-Brudenell: *Supporting Science, Design and Technology in the Early Years*
John Siraj-Blatchford and David Whitebread: *Supporting Information and Communications Technology Education in the Early Years*
Marian Whitehead: *Supporting Language and Literacy Development in the Early Years*

Supporting transitions in the early years

Liz *Brooker*

Open University Press

Open University Press
McGraw-Hill Education
McGraw-Hill House
Shoppenhangers Road
Maidenhead
Berkshire
England
SL6 2QL
email: enquiries@openup.co.uk
world wide web: www.openup.co.uk

and Two Penn Plaza, New York, NY 10121-2289, USA

First published 2008

A catalogue record of this book is available from the British Library

ISBN-10: 0-335-22168-8 (pb), 0-335-22169-6 (hb)
ISBN-13: 978-0-335-22168-4 (pb), 978-0-335-22169-1 (hb)

Library of Congress Cataloging-in-Publication Data
CIP data applied for

Typeset by YHT Ltd, London
Printed in Great Britain by Bell and Bain Ltd, Glasgow

The **McGraw·Hill** Companies

Contents

Acknowledgements

One of the pleasures of working towards this book over the last couple of years has been the discovery that I had joined a community of 'transitions researchers' that stretches around the world (and beyond the early years). It has been a great privilege to get to know them, and to learn from their experience. The community is large and elastic but among those I am most grateful to for their insights are Sue Dockett (Australia), Aline-Wendy Dunlop (Scotland), Hilary Fabian (England), Wilfred Griebel (Germany) and Sally Peters (New Zealand). Closer to home, I have benefited from the generosity of advisers and practitioners in English settings: Bernadette Duffy (Thomas Coram), Julie Fisher (then working for Oxfordshire), Caroline Pilcher and Liz Player (Norfolk) and Kathryn Solly (Chelsea Open Air Nursery); and from the insights of my talented students of transition: Rozanne Doyle, Katherine Hill, Glenda King, Gill Roberts and Lavinia Tiko.

The magic of electronic communication has brought a number of ex-students and other old and new acquaintances into the picture; their contribution was to listen to children's voices about transition, wherever they lived. I am very grateful to Maria Folque (Portugal), Sumaye Hamza (Nigeria), Rui Ma (China), Michelle McBean (Guyana), Mary O'Kane (Ireland), Ayako Shibata (Japan), Lavinia Tiko (Fiji) and Suborna Camellia (Bangladesh), and to Martin Woodhead who first gave me the idea of requesting their help.

Last but not least I wish to thank the many, many children, parents and teachers who have entrusted me with their experiences of young children's transitions.

Series editors' preface

This book is one of a series which will be of interest to all those who are concerned with the care and education of children from birth to 6 years old – childminders, teachers and other professionals in schools, those who work in playgroups, private and community nurseries and similar institutions; governors, providers and managers. We also speak to parents and carers, whose involvement is probably the most influential of all for children's learning and development.

Our focus is on improving the effectiveness of early education. Policy developments come and go, and difficult decisions are often forced on all those with responsibility for young children's well-being. We aim to help with these decisions by showing how developmental approaches to young children's education not only accord with our fundamental educational principles, but provide a positive and sound basis for learning.

Each book recognizes and demonstrates that children from birth to 6 years old have particular developmental learning needs, and that all those providing care and education for them would be wise to approach their work developmentally. This applies just as much to the acquisition of subject knowledge, skills and understanding, as to other educational goals such as social skills, attitudes and dispositions. In this series there are several volumes with a subject-based focus, and the main aim is to show how that can be introduced to young children within the framework of an integrated and developmentally appropriate curriculum, without losing its integrity as an area of knowledge in its own right. We also stress the importance of providing a learning environment which is carefully planned for children's own active learning.

Access for all children is fundamental to the provision of educational opportunity. We are concerned to emphasize anti-discriminatory approaches throughout, as well as the importance of recognizing that meeting special educational needs must be an integral purpose of curriculum development and planning. We see the role of play in learning as a central one, and one which also relates to all-round emotional, social and physical development. Play, along with other forms of active learning, is normally a natural point of access to the curriculum for each child at his or her particular stage and level of understanding. It is therefore an essential force in making for equal opportunities in learning, intrinsic as it is to all areas of development. We believe that these two aspects, play and equal opportunities, are so important that we not only highlight them in each volume in this series, but also include separate volumes on them as well.

Throughout this series, we encourage readers to reflect on the education being offered to young children, through revisiting the developmental principles which most practitioners hold, and using them to analyse their observations of the children. In this way, readers can evaluate ideas about the most effective ways of educating young children, and develop strategies for approaching their practice in ways which exemplify their fundamental educational beliefs, and offer every child a more appropriate education.

How all of the above beliefs and aspirations are to be achieved depends, of course, on the practices in homes and classrooms. But as this book shows, an important starting point is for children to settle satisfactorily and happily in the first instance. The way in which they are helped to move from one kind of provision to another is crucial here, and as the author makes abundantly clear, this affects not only early childhood, but matters throughout life.

The authors of each book in the series subscribe to the following set of principles for a developmental curriculum:

Principles for a developmental curriculum

- Each child is an individual and should be respected and treated as such.
- The early years are a period of development in their own right, and education of young children should be seen as a specialism with its own valid criteria of appropriate practice.
- The role of the educator of young children is to engage actively with

what most concerns the child, and to support learning through these preoccupations.

- The educator has a responsibility to foster positive attitudes in children to both self and others, and to counter negative messages which children may have received.
- Each child's cultural and linguistic endowment is seen as the fundamental medium of learning.
- An anti-discriminatory approach is the basis of all respect-worthy education, and is essential as a criterion for a developmentally appropriate curriculum (DAC).
- All children should be offered equal opportunities to progress and develop, and should have equal access to good quality provision. The concepts of multiculturalism and anti-racism are intrinsic to this whole educational approach.
- Partnership with parents should be given priority as the most effective means of ensuring coherence and continuity in children's experiences, and in the curriculum offered to them.
- A democratic perspective permeates education of good quality and is the basis of transactions between people.

Vicky Hurst and Jenefer Joseph

Introduction

Before this one I was at another school [a child development centre].
From that school my father brought me to this one. Now he's taking
me to another school. After I finish studying there he'll take me to
another big one. Then from that school I'll go to another one.

(Pre-school boy, aged 6, Bangladesh)

The entrance to a childcare centre, or to a nursery school, the tran-
sition from pre-school to school, from primary to secondary, from
secondary to tertiary or from school to work are some of the most
important phases and critical passings that compose a complex pro-
blem of education.

(Kavkoulis 1994: 42)

It is no accident that this book, which discusses young children's transitions, is in a series called *Supporting Early Learning*. The contexts in
which young children learn in modern societies are characterized,
overwhelmingly, by transitions of one kind or another, and everyone
who works with children has witnessed the impact that these transitions
can have on their learning, essentially through an impact on their well-
being. So this book has two overall aims: to explore, through examples of
research and practice, the ways that young children experience transitions in their daily lives, and to suggest the ways that the professional
expertise of practitioners can make the transition process a positive
learning experience, rather than a setback to learning. This introductory
chapter outlines some of the ways the topic is approached, some of the

themes that are addressed, and some of the questions the book attempts to answer.

One of its first tasks will be to consider the question, 'what do we mean by transitions?' Studies undertaken in this field over recent years have offered many answers. We will review the dimensions of transitions which are most commonly identified by researchers, and consider whether these descriptions apply to transitions in general, or just to the 'big one' that has traditionally occupied parents and practitioners – the start of formal, full-time school. At the same time we need to ask, 'what do we want from transitions?', in order to identify some shared understandings of the 'goals' of transition – other than simply getting it over with, as quickly as possible. We will consider too the question, 'why are transitions so important?', to establish why it is so essential to focus on the effects of change on children and families. And we will begin to consider the huge range of transitions that children may be required to make, in the days, weeks, months and years of early childhood. The nature of this range and variety is itself, of course, a reflection on the rapidly changing society we now inhabit.

Finally this chapter outlines the way that the book works, and the kinds of knowledge it builds on. The reader is introduced to the themes of each chapter and to the case studies of young children's transitions which are used to illustrate each of them. The case studies prompt a brief reflection on the nature of the research evidence available for anyone interested in transitions. The evidence comes from every continent, and it includes small studies focused on a single child, and large studies of 10,000 teachers. It is astonishing, in some ways, to see how much we already know about transitions, and disturbing, in other ways, to see how often this knowledge is disregarded as children make their transitions, from birth through to middle childhood.

What do we mean by transitions?

Transitions as a way of life

Transition has been a recognized characteristic of human lives, in every society we know of. In relatively simple pre-industrial societies, the naturally occurring changes in individual lives were often marked by ritual: not only birth and death but occasions such as the onset of puberty, the attainment of adulthood, or becoming a parent were marked, in families and communities, by feasts and ceremonies, special foods and special ornaments. Such rites of passage were a communal acknowledgement of events in the lives of individuals, and some of them would seem out of place in our own society, which views menstruation, for instance, as a private matter. But these developmental changes, whether public or private, shape all our lives, from a baby's first, dramatic entrance into the world through the many subsequent changes he or she experiences. All of us encounter, with varying degrees of pain and pleasure, the sensations of growing up and growing old, and all of us also experience the painful and pleasurable changes that occur in our relationships. The arrival of a younger sibling or the death or departure of a loved adult are also common experiences for children, while the birth of a child, or death of a partner, are life-changing events for us as adults. The ceremonies that accompany such events assure us that our family and community acknowledge and share our experiences.

In modern, complex societies, such events are more frequent and perhaps less regarded: as the dissolution and reconstitution of families becomes more common, society may appear to pay little attention to the lives of individuals. But for those involved, and especially for the youngest children, they may overturn all the predictability and security of daily life and make the world seem an unsafe and frightening place. Disruptions to relationships occur against a background of other changes: families move home more often, parents change jobs more often, and children may have multiple changes of caregiver. Many of the children in our schools and settings have lived through even bigger transitions, arriving in our villages, towns and cities as asylum seekers, refugees or economic migrants. The discontinuities such children have experienced in their earliest years – even before we meet them in a professional capacity – may be greater than their professional caregivers have experienced in the course of their own lives. So we may rarely meet a child, entering school for the first time, who has experienced the secure and stable early existence which was once viewed as the norm.

Rather than looking back nostalgically on a supposedly more stable age, we must remind ourselves of the positive aspects for children of growing up in the 21st century; of the constant opportunities to experience new ideas, to acquire new knowledge and skills, and to develop their own capacity for managing and making the most of new environments. We owe this optimistic outlook to the young children in our care. For them, the only certainty in life will be uncertainty, because the world they are inheriting, and in turn reshaping, is characterized by change. In the new millennium, it is clear, change is the default setting for our society, and the background for all the changes our children will experience as individuals.

Transitions into educational and care settings

One of the most significant consequences of social change for our young children is the shift from home to group care for children in their earliest years. As more and more women enter the workforce full time, it is now the norm in many societies for children to be placed in daycare before their first birthday (Neuman 2001). Although policies, practice and provision all vary from country to country (with a minority, like Finland, offering three years' maternity leave as an alternative to daycare), all post-industrial societies are moving towards a situation in which the majority of children experience some form of group care – whether regular full-day care or a weekly drop-in – long before the start of school. These early transitions require us to rethink, quite radically, the ways we view children's development, and their needs and rights, in infancy.

The diversity of this provision, and its significance for children, is further discussed in the next chapter. But in the UK, as in several other countries which have moved all services for young children under the auspices of an education ministry, children are now 'in education' for longer than at any time in human history. As the *Early Years Foundation Stage* is launched in England, children's daily lives will be regulated by Ofsted from shortly after their birth until they are 18 or older. Far from creating continuity, this provision could see them shift from daycare to pre-school and from nursery to reception class; from Foundation Stage unit to primary school, from primary to secondary, and from secondary to tertiary college. How many transitions is that? More importantly, are all these transitions planned and supported, or are some abrupt and scary? And what impact do they have on children's development and learning, their identity formation and their social competence?

Most of us have some vivid memories of particular transitions we have made within the education system, and some of us (including myself) have found the transitions we made as adults at least as alarming as those we remember from childhood. Research has identified the ways that transitions can threaten and undermine our sense of self-esteem, self-confidence and self-efficacy, and make us feel insecure and foolish. This may happen to us at any age, even if we have coped successfully with earlier transitions, so we can easily understand the vulnerability of children as their place in the world, and with it their sense of identity, is shaken up as they move from familiar to unfamiliar settings. At the same time we remind ourselves that all individuals are entitled to the chal-lenges and opportunities of 'lifelong learning', and that each time we make a good transition we may be starting on another intensely rewarding journey. So, 'good transitions' are the focus of this book.

Defining transitions

We will return to different ways of viewing transition, but we begin here with some important concepts which have helped to knit together the themes of this book.

First and foremost is the account of the 'father' of transition studies, Urie Bronfenbrenner, whose theoretical explanation of the transition process is introduced in Chapter 1. It was Bronfenbrenner's work with children and young families in the USA which triggered the huge 1960s early intervention programme, Project Head Start, and his understanding of the nature of transition, which permeated this particular project, resonates through all subsequent research. His description of the settings and relationships which make up the *ecological environment* is discussed later, but his definition of the transitions within this environment is both simple and comprehensive: a transition occurs when an individual's position in this environment 'is altered as the result of a change in role, setting, or both' (Bronfenbrenner 1979: 26). Children, in other words, are viewed not as isolated individuals but as *situated* in a social world, and any change in their environment (the settings in which they spend their days) will result in a change of role (the selfhood or identity they have constructed) which may have a significant and long-term impact on their development.

Bronfenbrenner's insights have shaped the direction of all subsequent research. Fthenakis (1998: 12), adopting his emphasis on role and identity, emphasizes that all transitions involve 'a reorganisation of roles', while Kagan and Neuman (1998: 366) define transitions as 'the continuity of experience that children have between periods and between spheres of their lives'. Fabian and Dunlop (2002: 3) opt to define transition as 'the process of change that is experienced when children (and their families) move from one setting to another', while a more recent account by Petriwskyj et al. (2005: 56) describes transition as 'an ongoing process of mutual adaptations by children, families and schools' to facilitate children's moves from setting to setting. All these terms – *processes, adaptations, continuities, roles, identities* – will play an important part in the discussion which follows, which sees all the changes in young children's lives as experiences which are shared by the child, family, peers and community.

This holistic understanding of transitions – as a process which includes all those involved in children's early lives – has not always been shared by policy makers, particularly in the USA, where large-scale transition studies have been funded by government. There, and in Australia (Petriwskyj 2005), transition strategies have concentrated on the concept of 'readiness', generally in the traditional sense of the 'readiness for school' of each individual child. The burden of responsibility for a successful transition, in this view, lies with the child and with those adults whose task it is to prepare her or him for 'stepping up' the educational ladder. Successful transitions, in this account, are achieved by individuals who have acquired the requisite academic knowledge and social skills to perform, conform and *learn* in the new setting. This perspective, which tends to blame those children, families and communities who have not achieved readiness, was exemplified in the first of the *US National Education Goals* ('by the year 2000, all children in America will start school ready to learn'; National Education Goals Panel 1991) although it has been repeatedly critiqued by researchers.

Why are transitions so important?

Transitions are a trigger for development and learning

Many of life's transitions, as suggested earlier, are inescapable, and all are for a purpose. Parents, as well as psychologists and educators, understand intuitively that children *need* change in order to develop. Parents who are interviewed before their children start pre-school, or when they make their move to school, or even to secondary school, always recognize that in some ways, and despite any apprehensions they may have, their children have outgrown their present environment and are 'ready to move on'. Rightly or wrongly, it is widely believed that 5-year-olds 'need' a different kind of stimulation from 4-year-olds in order to continue to develop; in the same way, 11-year-olds are thought to 'need' a much more strictly regulated and didactic learning environment than 10-year-olds.

Whether these age boundaries actually meet the developmental requirements of all children, or any children, is debatable, but the fact that transition into a new environment offers children a developmental trigger is not. Reception teachers, like parents, observe not only the intellectual sprint, but also the physical growth spurt, that seems to come from children's first encounter with school, as the short school haircuts turn into unruly mops, and the over-size clothes appear to rapidly shrink to fit the children inside them. And children's brain development in the early years accelerates as rapidly as their physical growth. Brain research in the last two decades has given us two important reminders. One is that the incessant growth of new synaptic connections in young children's brains is an almost unstoppable force which peaks during the pre-school years, but continues right into middle childhood and beyond (Shonkoff and Phillips 2000). The other is that this innate drive towards the expansion of brain capacity is both stimulated and sustained by the richness and variety of a child's environment, which can not only support the creation of new synapses, but equally importantly prevents the extinction of existing connections, which may occur if they are underused (Bruer 1999). It is understandable then that an environment which offers the ideal circumstances for small babies to develop their capacities may offer very few new stimuli for children of 3 or 5, who need novel experiences and challenges if they are to extend their thinking along new paths.

This 'developmental' aspect to transition experiences has been widely recognized for many years, but more recent research offers new arguments about the role of transitions in young children's lives and learning. Two important strands emerge from these new ways of thinking about children: the idea of learning as a *social* rather than a *solitary* (or individual) activity, and the idea of 'learning dispositions', rather than knowledge and skills, as the most important goals for early learning.

Learning and knowledge are social and situated

Knowledge and skills have traditionally been viewed as attributes of individuals, which could be 'measured' or 'tested' and found to be either present or absent in a particular child. The history of IQ testing is the best-known example of this view: it assumed that children could be assigned a number, or placed in a category, which defined their intelligence in terms of certain measurable abilities such as understanding a two-part instruction, or answering a question about 'which is greater?', or naming a letter or number or object.

Early years educators have never been sympathetic to this view of children's learning, and there have been numerous challenges to it over the last half-century. These challenges began perhaps with the discovery that children's success in the 11-plus exam – taken by all children in the UK until a few decades ago – had more to do with their social class background than with their so-called 'intelligence' (and that many 11-plus 'failures' went on to become intellectual leaders). They continued with the groundbreaking research of those like Donaldson (1978) and Tizard and Hughes (1984) who showed that children's ability to succeed in school-like test situations bore little relation to their abilities in everyday contexts. Donaldson and her colleagues showed that children who 'failed' various Piagetian tasks could accomplish them easily when they were reworded as meaningful tasks for the children involved. At the

same time, Tizard and Hughes, and Wells (1985), were offering con-
clusive evidence that children who appeared to be inarticulate or
uncomprehending in their classroom interactions could display ample
mastery of language and conceptual thinking in their conversations with
family members at home. By now it was clear that children's knowledge,
skills and abilities were not just 'there' in the child, to be identified and
assessed, but were present in children's social practices, in their meaningful interactions with the world, and in their relationships. In other
words, children's ability to demonstrate their knowledge and apply their
skills is a function of their social environment, and of their own sense of
belonging within that environment. The question to be asked is not, 'do
they know it or don't they?' but 'are they able to apply their knowledge
in this setting?', a very different matter.

The view of learning as social and situated reflects an understanding of
the major role played by children's social development – their confidence, self-esteem and sense of self-efficacy – in their continuing
cognitive development. Like adults, children can be hampered in their
ability to think clearly and act competently when they are feeling insecure or vulnerable, and their development may slow down or stop if they
remain in this insecure condition for very long. Yet it is often in their first
days and weeks in a new setting – in the actual process of transition –
that early assessments of them are made, if only informally. Identifying
transition as first and foremost a social process is an important step
towards supporting children's learning in their early days in a new
environment.

Transitions are an opportunity to strengthen positive dispositions

In addition to the traditionally valued – and easily taught, and tested –
components of early learning, such as knowledge (colours, shapes,
numbers, letters) and skills (cutting, tying, sticking, fastening),
researchers have identified attributes which may have a far greater long-
term impact on children's lives: learning dispositions, or attitudes of
mind. These dispositions are the attributes which may not only *support*
transitions, but be strengthened and fostered *by* transitions

Like the potential for brain growth, dispositions to learn are believed
to be innate in children, but also capable of being strengthened or
extinguished through early experiences. They consist more of an attitude
of mind – an attitude to oneself, to one's life and to one's learning – than
of any acquired knowledge or skills. Lillian Katz (1994) was one of the
first early childhood experts to develop a comprehensive account of what

dispositions are, where they come from, and why they are important. In doing so she makes a powerful case for focusing on dispositions as the main goal or outcome of early learning. We should focus on dispositions, in Katz's view, for a number of reasons, including these:

- The mere acquisition of knowledge and skills does not mean that they will be used and applied. Listening skills do not make children listen, and reading skills do not make children read: children need also to feel *disposed* to listen or to read.
- Instruction in skills may actually undermine the disposition to use those skills: 'drill' in reading may tend to discourage children from reading.
- Some innate dispositions, such as the urge to investigate, need to be carefully encouraged because they may be extinguished during formal education.
- Dispositions can not be acquired through direct instruction but must be modelled for children by those around them, for instance, by teachers who 'think aloud' about the best way to do things.

Increasingly powerful arguments for the role of dispositions in learning have been made in the last few years. Margaret Carr (2001), co-author of the New Zealand early years curriculum *Te Whaariki*, has argued eloquently for a focus on certain key dispositions in both the pre-school and the school experience. The dispositions she looks for in her work with children include 'taking an interest' and 'persisting with difficulty', and her explanation of the factors which enable children to be 'ready, willing and able' to learn is a thread which underpins this book.

Transitions may have long-lasting effects

One of the unfortunate aspects of previous research on transitions is that so much of the evidence points to the long-term as well as short-term problems caused by difficult or unhappy transitions. Once again, research in different national contexts has focused on different issues. The large-scale transition studies conducted in the USA from the 1970s onwards stemmed from a concern that the benefits of early interventions, like Head Start, 'washed out' or faded once children were in school. National projects such as the Head Start Transition Project (Hubbell et al. 1987) and the National Transition Study (Love et al. 1992) aimed to identify what children and their families needed to know by the time the child started school, or in other words to identify the components of 'readiness'.

Because of the scale of these studies, which involved thousands of children, parents and teachers, only the broadest of categories could be analysed: children in rural, urban or suburban areas; children from two-parent or one-parent families; children from minority ethnic or white families. The significant influences on their transition were equally broadly delineated, and included the relative benefits of a focus on social development, or on school rules, or on 'academics', in the home or pre-school. The most evident finding from studies of this kind was that the children categorized as having the fewest home advantages – those from poor, black, inner-city neighbourhoods – received the least support for their transition to elementary school, and made the least progress over the first three school grades, so that the benefits of their pre-school experience soon faded. This evident waste of a national investment in early learning prompted the development of a number of transition frameworks designed to sustain the positive outcomes of pre-school for children.

Studies in the UK and Europe have typically been smaller in scale, and have focused more on the ways that social and emotional difficulties during transition have impacted on children's continuing development and learning. Early studies by Hughes et al. (1979), Jackson (1979) and Cleave et al. (1982) considered the affective nature of transitions, and the ways that children's fears of the unknown, or their ignorance of school rules and cultures, or their unhappiness over separation, created long-term insecurities and barriers to learning.

These studies, taken together, suggested that a minority of children, perhaps from 5 to 10 per cent, adapted poorly to school and continued to be at risk of school failure as a result, potentially creating a huge pool of unhappy children and unfulfilled adults.

What are the goals of transition?

Promoting well-being and belonging

A fundamental goal of a school-start transition is to help young children feel *suitable* in school, that is, to have a feeling of well-being and belonging.

(Broström 2002: 52)

The positive learning dispositions discussed earlier have been described as the most important outcome of early learning (Sylva 1994), and I have argued that they should be viewed as an important outcome of transitions. But there is an even broader agenda here, one which is best described as *well-being*, a term which we can view as the short-term and the long-term goal of all our work with children, and an over-arching goal for our support for transitions.

Well-being as a total condition – physical, social, emotional, intellectual – was the label given by a powerful group of early educators and researchers to the experiences of children in the *Experiential Education* and *Effective Early Learning* studies (Pascal and Bertram 1997; Laevers and Heylen 2003). It is defined by Ferre Laevers – the founder, with colleagues, of the *Experiential Education* project – as a state in which children are fully involved and absorbed in their chosen activities, supported by sensitive adults who ensure their autonomy. Laevers and his colleagues recognized that children's involvement could be described in ways that made it possible to compare settings as well as children, and so to identify what kinds of environmental and adult support enabled children to reach high levels of well-being.

Although the specific focus here, as in Laevers' work, is on children's *learning*, this is inseparable from the broader notion of well-being which is encompassed in the Framework for Children's Services in England, *Every Child Matters* (DfES 2003). The Framework is built on five outcomes for children, including physical health and emotional security, enjoying and achieving, making a contribution, and avoiding poverty. All are viewed as essential components of well-being. As many studies have demonstrated, successful 'learning' in the early years is only likely to occur when children's physical and emotional needs are met: Myers (1992), Woodhead (1996) and others have shown that in many parts of the world a nutrition programme is the most important preparation for school. Though relatively few children in western societies are seriously undernourished, it is understood that anyone working with young children must maintain a watchful eye on their physical as well as their social and emotional development, all of which sustain their cognitive learning.

Emotional and social well-being are conjured up very well both by Carr's (2001) concept of 'belonging', one of the key dispositions of *Te Whaariki*, and by Broström's notion of feeling 'suitable', a state children achieve 'when they successfully negotiate the daily challenges of kindergarten life, including both social (peer-related) and academic (content-related) challenges' (2002: 52). This important state is also represented by Laevers (1997) – in a borrowed phrase – as being like 'fish in water', an image which is exemplified in some of the case studies discussed in later chapters.

Achieving the 3 Rs

Gordon Wells and Guy Claxton (2002), who advocate the importance of
early learning as a foundation for life-long learning, identify certain key
qualities as fundamental to learning, and these are similar to those
identified by Gillian Pugh (2002) in her advocacy of investment in services for young children. These key characteristics go under different
names, but one way of conveying them is through labels such as *resilience*
(persisting through difficulties), *resourcefulness* (solving problems) and
reciprocity (acting collaboratively and constructively with others).

These three terms – 3 Rs, but with a very different emphasis from the
Rs we grew up with – enable us to understand many aspects of children's transitions, and I will return to them throughout the book.
Transition experiences sometimes seem to remove these attributes from
children, making them more helpless and dependent, less confident and
pro-social. But I will argue that this need not be the case, and that well-
supported transitions serve to strengthen children's resilience and
resourcefulness, and enhance their reciprocity, so that they are better
equipped for the changing future ahead of them. A successful transition
should result in a child who feels strong and competent, and able to
handle new experiences with confidence. These are the children described by Carr (2001) as *ready, willing and able* to learn – a different kind of
readiness than is sometimes expected of children.

How the book is organized

My aims in this book, as I explained, are twofold: to explore our
understanding of young children's transitions, and at the same time to
identify the best ways to support them through the experience, so that
with each successive 'move' they can acquire greater resilience,
resourcefulness and reciprocity. In keeping with the principles of the
Every Child Matters agenda, I consider both the type of support that is
needed for 'all children', and also the additional support that may be
needed by more vulnerable children. This group may include children
with Special Educational Needs (1 in 5 of all children at some stage of
their education, but possibly 100% of all children on their first day in a
new setting); children from minority ethnic backgrounds including those
with English as an Additional Language; and children whose family
circumstances may require them to make more frequent, more sudden or
more difficult transitions throughout their educational career. Although I
refer throughout the book to international research and practice, most of

my examples, and the case studies, are from English settings, the location for my own experiences as a teacher and researcher.

The next chapter focuses on the diverse experiences of early childhood, and the range and diversity of early transitions, as well as introducing key theories for understanding how transitions affect children. It is followed, in Chapter 2, by a discussion of the early transitions made by babies and toddlers, and then in Chapter 3 by an exploration of the different 'cultures' of homes and schools. Chapter 4 deals with the continuities and discontinuities experienced as children 'move up' within the education system, while Chapter 5 is given over to evidence of children's own perspectives on their pre-schools and schools, and the transitions between them. Finally, Chapter 6 looks at the role of assessment in shaping children's transition experiences and their development as learners, while Chapter 7 considers the lessons learned about supporting and strengthening children's resilience, resourcefulness and reciprocity as they move into middle childhood.

Each of these chapters offers case studies of individual children, nurseries, classrooms, schools or LEAs as examples of the transition experience. Many of the examples come from my own work as a practitioner and as a researcher, but I am grateful too to the colleagues, including my students, who have offered their own evidence. Their studies address both the move from home into group care, and subsequent moves between phases. They include evidence on starting school in Ireland, moving from nursery to Reception in London, moving from pre-school to Primary School in Fiji, moving from pre-school to Primary 1 in Northern Ireland, moving from pre-school to Reception for 'gifted and talented' children and for children with learning difficulties, and moving from the Foundation Stage to Year 1.

These studies are all relatively small in scale; some were undertaken by a single researcher, though others used a team of practitioners, and each has investigated a small sample of participants – children, parents, teachers and teacher-trainers. They serve to highlight, not only the different perspectives there can be on transition, but the different types of research which are referred to in this book. The transitions 'literature' includes studies of 3500 schools and 10,000 kindergarten teachers (Rimm-Kaufman et al. 2000, USA) and studies of six schools with six different ethnic groups (Dockett and Perry 2005, Australia) as well as studies of just 50 children (Fabian 1996, UK) or three (Dalli 2000, New Zealand). All are significant, because each study has asked an important question about the experience of transition, and has attempted to answer it honestly and comprehensively. Without small-scale studies we could not hope to hear the voices of individual children; without large-scale studies we would not have a context for these individual voices. In presenting findings from both approaches I have tried to explain my own understanding of children's transitions, and of the ways these can be supported.

1

Understanding early transitions: more than 'starting school'

I was looking forward to go to pre-school for the first time. When I always pass the pre-school centre, I always tell my mother that I am old and that I need to be at pre-school. My mother says no because I am too young, I'm still a baby. I replied that I am not drinking milk any longer. I am a big girl now, and I needed to go to school.

(Pre-school girl, Fiji)

Children, like adults, enjoy and are stimulated by novelty and change. The first day of school, the transfer to 'big school', are landmarks in the process of growing up. Even when children are apprehensive, they look forward to change ... But if change is to stimulate and not to dishearten, it must be carefully prepared and not too sudden.

(*Plowden Report*, 1967)

Life has changed a great deal in the last 50 years, and the first day of 'big school' may no longer be such a developmental milestone for children as it was for their parents and grandparents, in the days when Lady Plowden and her committee were conducting their interviews. This chapter examines some of the changes in policy and provision for under-5s that have occurred over the last few decades, and asks whether the Plowden committee's account is still relevant in today's world – for children starting school, or for all early transitions. It also introduces aspects of the most widely used theory of transitions, Bronfenbrenner's account of the 'ecological environment' within which we all live and grow. Like all good theories, Bronfenbrenner's is a key to good practice, helping us to see both why children's experiences are so varied, and how we can make them better.

I begin with the stories of Joshua and Jelika, two of the 4-year-olds who started school, in a multicultural classroom, at All Saints' Primary (Brooker 2002).

Case study: Joshua

Joshua's birthday was in August, and he started school in September as a very young 4-year-old, as a consequence of the LEA's single-point-of-entry policy. He was small in comparison with other children in his Reception class, and appeared rather quiet and watchful during his first sessions in the classroom. Within days however he was observed chatting merrily with his teacher and nursery nurse, relaying long stories about his cousins and his dog (his punch-line, 'So that's funny, isn't it?' reduced them to near-tears of laughter after a while) and informing them of precisely what he had in mind to do today ('*First*, right, I'm going to have a little go at those popoids ... *then* I might go outside with Katy – if she wants to ...'). His quiet confidence, and sense of belonging, became evident in every move he made. He was *suitable* in the setting.

The secret of Joshua's successful transition lay in his earlier experiences – at home, in group care and in relation to the school. His dad was a long-distance lorry-driver and often away from home, but his mum, Maisie, had taken a playgroup leader's qualification, and helped to run the playgroup in a nearby community hall. Joshua had attended playgroup several mornings a week, 'unofficially', since he was tiny, and knew many of the children who had moved up from the same group. But he had also experienced a range of equivalent experiences at home: Maisie was an enthusiast for collage and playdough, Lego and Duplo, paints and puzzles, and offered Joshua a rich diet of talking and sharing books while his older sisters were at school in the afternoons. Joshua could have explained to some of his new class-mates, who had a very different pre-school experience, exactly what you were supposed to do with many of the activities on display.

In the process of bringing and collecting his two big sisters, Joshua had also been an apprentice, on a daily basis, to this business of 'going to school': he knew the layout of the building and the playgrounds, the routines for dropping off reading books and selecting new ones, the ways that adults were greeted and talked to, and something of the limits to the friendly informality that pervaded the school – the boundaries that could not be crossed. His 'transition' did not begin on the day he started in September, nor on the day of his 'visit' in June: he had been 'starting school' for most of his life, so that when the day finally came, the reality of being left to fend for himself in a large group of his peers for several hours came as only a slight shock. Most importantly, he had already identified the adults in the classroom as friendly beings, on first-name terms with his mum, with whom one could have a relaxed relationship.

Starting school at All Saints': one classroom, many experiences

Joshua's social identity was well matched to his new classroom, and required only small adjustments: to a great extent he could be *himself* in the setting. Because he started school fully equipped with school-like resources, and confident in making relationships, his resilience was not tested by the experience. Other children studied in the same classroom were less fortunate, and comparing aspects of Joshua's situation with theirs makes the reasons very clear. Among the 16 children whose transitions were observed, the following characteristics had an identifiable impact:

- Eight children had learned English as their first language, while eight had grown up speaking Sylheti.
- Eight had mothers who had attended primary school in England, while seven had attended in Bangladesh and one had never been to school.
- Three children were the oldest in their family, while others were the second, third, fourth or sixth sibling.
- Eight of the children had pre-school experience of group care, although one of these 'only went twice', and other twins 'soon gave up because they cried'; three were playgroup regulars like Joshua, and two had attended an integrated nursery centre.
- Twelve of the children had older siblings in the school.
- Four of the children had a mother who had herself been permanently excluded from school as a teenager.
- Six of the children lived in households without a regular wage-earner.

There are no simple connections, of course, between any of these 'home' characteristics and a child's experiences of starting school. But cumulatively, as the All Saints' study showed, they may contribute to life-styles which are *more* or *less* like the learning environment of the classroom; to adult–child relationships which *more* or *less* resemble those offered by teachers; to expectations and demands which match, or conflict with, those of schools (Brooker 2002). Some aspects of children's early lives – poverty, family illness, maternal depression, stress, intimidation, social exclusion – were written into their bodies as well as their minds by the time they entered the welcoming environment of the reception class. Some households, through no fault of their own, had barely been able to secure the basic rights to health care, nutrition, adequate clothing and the experience of a 'family' for their small children. Starting school did not wipe out these inequalities.

Early education, and early childhood services in general, have historically and more recently been designed to redress some of the household inequalities which construct social exclusion in children's lives. By the age of 4, some of the children now growing up in the UK are in urgent need of an environment that is rich in opportunities. Their transition into that new environment may shape the direction of their learning journey for many years to come, so getting it right is extremely important. Understanding theory can help us to do so, as we will see in relation both to Joshua's story and to that of his classmate Jelika.

Case study: Jelika

Jelika started school in the same week and in the same classroom as Joshua but her transition experience was as different from his as it could be. Pollard has pointed out that 'each child experiences the classroom in the light of their particular structural position, learning stance, interests, strategies, identity and cultural background' (Pollard with Filer 1996: 281), and Jelika's background had not prepared her for an easy transition. Now aged 4, she had arrived from Bangladesh with her parents as an infant, and moved into her grandparents' house, where she spent her days in the company of relatives of all ages, including her teenage aunties and her two younger brothers. She had never attended any kind of preschool, and her mother had warned the Bangladeshi assistant, in the course of a home visit, that Jelika was very frightened of going to school because she had 'never seen so many people together', and 'never met any English people'.

For Jelika the transition process began, very abruptly, on her first day of school. Her mother, who spoke no English, appeared as nervous as her daughter as she delivered her to the classroom door for her first half-day session in September. On that occasion, as no meaningful verbal exchange was possible, her kindly teacher led her by the hand to where three other Bangladeshi girls were standing, in the home corner, and encouraged them to play together. But Jelika's strategy, in the face of her evident fears, appeared to be a kind of heroic stoicism. My field notes from that afternoon report: 'Jelika stood rigid and unsmiling all afternoon, hands at her sides, eyes straight ahead; refused to touch or play with anything, or listen to the Bengali story [the bilingual assistant was called in for this]; didn't actually cry; other Bengali children totally ignored her'.

The other three girls, though less anxious than Jelika, were also rather bewildered by their new environment, and preferred to cling to the safety of the threesome they had already forged. In the following days my field notes report: 'Jelika is silent, but doesn't seem to be actually frightened or distressed. I asked Tuhura, Rufia and Khiernssa if they would talk to her but they all said no'. It was left to Jelika to summon the resources to manage her own transition, which she did. On her fourth day she 'began to smile and laugh', the following day witnessed her first attempts at verbal communication, and only a week later, while happily playing outdoors, she began chatting to two Bengali boys.

Over her first term, my observations revealed the range of her self-help strategies:

- She enlisted me [classroom researcher rather than teacher] as her individual tutor, leading me to activities and requesting demonstrations and assistance to enable her to participate.
- She practised unfamiliar skills over and over to gain mastery.
- She looked, listened and carefully imitated the monolingual children: she soon began to interpret, using gestures, for the two little boys, tactfully eliciting their needs and trying to communicate them to non-Bengali speakers.
- She 'adopted' another child, Tuhura, and acted as her mentor, guide and mother-figure in the classroom.

Though unable to find a role in the mainstream life of the classroom, she had created her own small Bangladeshi peer group, with its own membership (mostly female) and its own routines and rituals. By the end of term she was a happy and relaxed participant in this group, though she remained a very peripheral participant in the class as a whole.

These observations suggest that Jelika, by calling on her own inner resources and dispositions, accomplished her transition to school with very little support from others. In her first term she had taken one huge step – from the familiar world of home to a secure world of her peers – but she needed still to take the further steps which would integrate her into the culture of the class as a whole, and of her teachers. This was essential because that mainstream culture was the 'learning culture' through which children could access the knowledge and skills they needed to succeed in school. When she was assessed by teachers on entry, her cognitive scores were among the highest for the Bengali children, which placed her on a level with the lowest-achieving monolingual children. Sadly, she was awarded very low 'scores' in the baseline assessment of Personal, Social and Emotional development, and her scores on each of the component scales (such as 'initiative', 'relationships', 'cooperation' and 'involvement') indicated that she had not shown herself to be a very 'suitable' participant in the classroom.

Understanding early transitions: theoretical perspectives

While there have been many attempts to define and describe the transition experience – as a process of separation and attachment, of loss and gain, of rites of passage – the theoretical explanation that researchers and practitioners have found most helpful is Bronfenbrenner's.

Bronfenbrenner, as well as being hailed as the 'father of Head Start', is widely known for his ecological theory of human development, which describes the human individual as a participant in an array of interlocking 'systems', all of which have an impact, either direct or indirect, on his or her development. Bronfenbrenner's major study, *The Ecology of Human Development* (1979) discusses evidence from every stage of the life-cycle in support of his argument: mothers and babies in neo-natal units, children starting school, adolescents getting in and out of risky situations, mental health patients in institutions, and old people in care homes. For every stage and every group he is able to demonstrate the extent to which the *links* between the various systems one person experiences enable that person's transitions *between* the systems to be effective and positive, rather than detrimental and negative.

The applications of this theory to young children's transitions are very clear. Bronfenbrenner's explanations are equally helpful when applied to individual cases – children – or to policies and practices adopted more broadly. Each setting the child experiences – home, childminder's house, granny's house, nursery, or school – is described as a *microsystem,* and each of these has a role to play in the child's development. But Bronfenbrenner argues that the most important contribution to a child's well-being is the set of links between the microsystems – which he calls a *mesosystem.* Basically, the more links there are, and the stronger these links are, the better the child's experience and outcomes are likely to be, as this 'proposition' asserts:

> The developmental potential of a setting is increased as a function of the number of supportive links existing between that setting and other settings (such as home and family). Thus the least favourable condition for development is one in which supplementary links are either non-supportive or completely absent, when the mesosystem is weakly linked.
>
> (Bronfenbrenner 1979: 215)

Informal meetings between parents and teachers offer face-to-face links, which may be strengthened by home visits from the teacher or time spent in the classroom by the parent. At another level, links may consist of forms that provide information about the child's preferences and routines (information from home to school), or letters and messages sent by the teacher, or on behalf of the school or setting (information from setting to home). At the child's own level, familiar objects carried to and fro between home and school may offer security in an unfamiliar environment.

Some of Bronfenbrenner's 'hypotheses' are clearly exemplified in the good practice of many schools and settings, for instance: 'Upon entering a new setting, the person's development is enhanced to the extent that valid information, advice and experience relevant to one setting are made available, on a continuing basis, to the other' (1979: 217).

Even more important than this exchange of information, of course, is the actual presence of a parent or friend from home while the child is settling. In Bronfenbrenner's terms, 'The developmental potential of a setting in a mesosystem is enhanced if the person's initial transition into that setting is not made alone' (1979: 211). But he makes clear too that this one-off transition event is not a sufficient link, and that the continuation of links between all parts of the mesosystem is essential. When children are young, it may seem as if the 'transition' from one microsystem to another takes place daily, or at least weekly, and is felt especially acutely after a break or holiday, so the supportive links between home and school need to be constantly available, and constantly renewed. Perhaps this aspect, rather than simply the initial transition and settling, is something that practitioners need to be aware of.

Bronfenbrenner's explanation confirms what common sense tells us about Joshua and Jelika. For the former, the links between home and school had been constructed since infancy, and were continually re-established as his mother brought him into the classroom every day. His development, accordingly, went from strength to strength. For the latter, no such links had existed in the pre-school years, and none were constructed during her transition.

'Landmarks in the process of growing up'

When the *Plowden Report* (CACE 1967) first coined this phrase, very little was known, except anecdotally, about children's experience of transitions. Since then, research into transitions has tracked the changes in children's early experiences as well as in the ways that transition is viewed by parents, practitioners and policy makers – only recently have the views of the children themselves been taken into account, as we will see in Chapter 5. In England, the earliest studies of transition examined, from very different perspectives, the experience and consequences of starting school at 5 (Hughes et al. 1979; Jackson 1979). Hughes and his colleagues were prompted by their observations of children's tears and distress on starting school to follow up these 'difficult' transitions and see what impact they had on children's subsequent experience, while Jackson chose to enter imaginatively into the minds of children from diverse family backgrounds, to show what school looked like, felt like and smelt like to each of them. Before long, more comprehensive studies were published, reflecting the changing realities of children's lives. They demonstrated both how children experienced the 'first transition', from home to pre-school (Blatchford et al. 1982), and then the move from pre-school to primary school (Cleave et al. 1982; Barrett 1986). These latter volumes identified in quite chilling detail the range of factors that could contribute to making children's early days at school either exhilarating or excruciating. But by then the provision offered to children before the start of school was itself undergoing rapid change.

Transitions over the last half-century: the rise of pre-school provision

Although the rapid pace of change in the 21st century has become a cliché, it is still important to ask whether our policies and procedures always reflect and incorporate such change as it occurs. In terms of transition, for instance, does 'starting school' still represent a landmark in children's lives, or is it now just one step in a long sequence of steps from birth to adulthood? And are our current policies, provision and practice based on ideas derived from our own early experiences (or those of our own children) rather than on the lived experiences of young children today?

In England as in other countries, the change process appears to accelerate from the 1960s, a decade already labelled by history as the era of child-centred philosophies and the flowering of English primary education (Pluckrose 1987). The 1960s were also an era when few children were offered more than a few hours a week of group care before they started school. Many of the nursery schools that were opened during the Second World War had closed down in the late 1940s, and the playgroup movement, the brainchild of middle-class mothers, was in its earliest infancy. Only the most privileged in society (those who could pay for private nursery schools) and the least privileged (those whose children were taken off to Social Services nurseries for their own good) had guaranteed access to under-5 provision. The statutory school starting date, as now, was the term after the child's fifth birthday, and many children spent the years from birth to 5 at home or in family care, except for the odd afternoon at a toddler group or crèche. This simple sequence – home from birth to 5; then school after your fifth birthday – was soon to change, propelled by demographic changes of many kinds.

The blossoming of playgroup provision in the UK was a grass-roots response to changing circumstances, which produced mothers who wanted to get out of the home, and also wanted their children to experience peer companionship and play opportunities before school. A further spur to extending pre-school provision during the 1970s was the realization, at government and local authority level, that declining birth rates had left many schools with falling rolls and empty classrooms; classrooms that could be profitably turned into rooms for 3- and 4-year-olds, thus increasing the school's roll, preparing children for primary school, and recruiting them for a longer-term place in the school (Bennett and Kell 1989). The gradual downward age trend, caused by the falling birth rate and its impact on school finances, meant that by the 1990s most children started in reception classes soon after their fourth birthday, despite the persistence of an official school start date a whole year later (Woodhead 1989; Dowling 1995).

By contrast, the simultaneous expansion of pre-school education in the USA represented a top-down intervention on a colossal scale, and in non-school settings. In the mid 1960s, Project Head Start was launched, offering pre-school provision before kindergarten with the express purpose of intervening in the cycle of deprivation which produced poor academic and social outcomes for children from poor families, in both inner-city and rural districts (Vinovskis 2005). Forty years later, millions of children still routinely enrol in Head Start programmes every year (and millions of words of research have written about the impact of these programmes). At the same time, statutory schooling still begins with First Grade, rather than kindergarten, in many American states, and the compulsory age for school entrance remains high and variable: 'entry to formal elementary school is generally not mandated until children reach the age of six to eight years' (Gill et al. 2006). So despite some superficial similarities, including a heavy reliance on private providers, a wide gulf of differences separates the early years provision in the UK and the USA, and the process of starting school in one society may bear little resemblance to a comparable process in the other.

By the end of the 1990s the majority of children in advanced industrial societies were accessing some form of pre-school provision, from the age of 3 until the start of school.

Towards the 21st century: accommodating under-3s

By the 1990s too, the under-3s revolution was already sneaking up on us. More and more women in many countries wished to, or were obliged to, begin work when their children were under 3 years old, resulting in a huge expansion and diversity of services. In England, by the time the Conservative government left office in 1997, children were experiencing a kaleidoscope of provision, from short term to full day, and from excellent to awful, before they started in Reception in the months before their fifth birthday. This provision included:

- Nursery schools (LEA) and nursery classes in primary schools.
- Integrated and family centres.
- Playgroups and pre-schools (voluntary and private).
- Private nursery and pre-prep schools.
- Crèches, drop-ins and 'mums & tots' at community venues.
- Childminding.
- Family care.

Two important events, coinciding with the election of a Labour government in 1997, promised to give more coherence to this hotch-potch: in policy terms, the launch of Early Years Development and Childcare Partnerships (EYDCPs), which obliged local authorities to audit and monitor and regulate their provision for under-5s; and in research terms, the launch of the Effective Provision of Pre-school Education (EPPE) project, whose vast database was to create a much clearer picture of what was going on, at least for 3–5-year-olds, in the UK.

The EYDCPs were the first step in a longer-term programme of providing and regulating childcare at a more central level, with the intention of safeguarding children's rights to quality care, and ensuring that the entitlement reached all corners of society. A succession of new initiatives propelled more and more children into early experiences of group care, as tax credits (enabling parents to pay for child care out of their earnings) began to replace the benefits which encouraged parents to remain at home, and as overall social policies emphasized the importance of paid employment in combating social exclusion and family poverty. No sooner was the Foundation Stage curriculum for 3- and 4-year-olds in place (DfES/QCA 2000), than the government turned its attention to the neglected area of 0–3 provision. With the publication of *Birth to Three Matters* (DfES 2002) the education and care of the youngest children became a public responsibility even if it was a private arrangement. Children's first steps on the road to school were now, officially, taken in the early months of their lives.

Multiple provision – multiple transitions

Interim reports from the EPPE project soon revealed what children were actually experiencing in the years before they started school, as the study analysed interviews with parents, which tracked the early, birth-to-3, experiences of each of the 3500 children involved. The statistics produced in the early years of the project lent substance to what many practitioners had already identified: the actuality of *horizontal,* as well as *vertical,* transitions.

Where transitions have traditionally meant 'stepping up' the ladder to the next stage of schooling, the EPPE findings demonstrated that many young children were also 'stepping sideways' in their experiences of group care. Parents who needed to work or study were frequently obliged to make complicated arrangements for their young children's care: off early in the morning to a relative or childminder, and then on again into a half-day nursery or pre-school; back to the childminder, out to a toddler group, and back to the childminder or relative to await the parent's return. Even if each of the settings a child experiences is suitable and appropriate, safe and secure, the child's cumulative experience of changes, within the day or within the week, is both unplanned and unprecedented. Similar findings emerge from a slightly earlier US study (Mangione and Speth 1998) which argues the need to strike a balance between what the authors call *horizontal and vertical continuity,* where horizontal continuities are the links between the services a child is experiencing at one point in time, and vertical continuities are the links between services experienced over time. And, as Petriwskyj et al. (2005) point out, an additional set of transitions is added where children are identified as having special needs, and are offered specialized care and services on top of their mainstream provision. These children, who may be less able to comprehend and control their own daily experiences than typically developing children, may actually be faced with even more challenges than their peers.

What are the alternatives to such multiple transitions? Different societies offer different solutions, but there is little hard evidence to show what is in children's best interests. Does the universally available, well-funded, full-day care offered in some Scandinavian countries offer the best solution? It is tempting to think so, but then where do we draw the line in providing non-stop care? (For me, this question was prompted by talking to Finnish practitioners who work in '24-hour' nurseries, where some small children stay from Monday morning to Friday evening, going home to spend the weekend with their parents). Does the offer of maternal leave for 36 months (also in Finland, but at some financial sacrifice for parents) offer a better alternative? Should parents be able to choose, freely, whether to stay at home, go to work or study, or combine the two in the way that meets their own needs? Most importantly, are parents' needs and babies' needs identical? It is likely that, at different moments in a child's early years, they are not. In such instances, the rights of babies, or at least their preference for a calm environment and consistency of care, may be sacrificed to the needs or wishes of their parents.

Meanwhile, at the present moment, young children in the UK and elsewhere may be delivered from one location to another in the course of a single day, setting the practitioners who care for them the challenge of providing the security and continuity which supports their well-being. And in consequence, our understanding of 'transitions' as special occasions, 'landmarks in the process of growing up', which we can plan for, celebrate and support, may need some adjustment.

Starting school: at 6, 5 or 4?

The age at which children make their 'big transition' into statutory schooling has always been controversial. In the UK, the statutory age of 5 was decided in 1870, and has remained the same, while practice has gradually drawn children in up to a year earlier (Woodhead 1989).

Meanwhile, in many parts of the world, the statutory requirement to be in school is much later, and the 'pre-school' period may constitute a relaxed and playful experience which some of our own children might envy.

Are there any 'good', developmental, reasons why this is so? The UK starting age was decided long before the child study movement, and the developmental psychologists, had identified any age-related stages in children's development. As Bertram and Pascal point out, the UK decision 'related to the exigencies of a political compromise agreed in the House of Commons in the 1860s, and had no rational basis in educational theory' (2002: 9). These authors remind us too that before the 1870 Act, 'it was not uncommon to find two-year-olds in formal church and secular schools ... especially in rural areas at harvest times or industrialized areas such as Lancashire where large numbers of women were employed' (2002: 9). The practical expediency which prompted the emergence of 'infant schools' and 'babies' classes' in 19th-century England has prompted many of the subsequent changes in legislation and practice regarding young children's education and care: these include the opening of state nurseries in 1940 (to release mothers for war work), the closure of these nurseries after 1945 (to allow men to return to their civilian employment) and the opening of nursery classes in the 1980s (to fill the vacancies created by a declining birth rate). In response, many of our beliefs about 'ages and stages' seem to have evolved to fit the reality, so that for most parents – if not for practitioners – 5 seems the 'right' age to be starting school, and the practice in other countries of enrolling children at 6 or 7 seems a little odd.

In Europe, for instance, Norway has only recently brought its school-entry age down from 7 to 6 (with a 'pre-school' year of informal activities); Finnish children are in informal daycare until they are 6, with a 'pre-school' year that includes some academic input; while Italian, French and German children too start school at 6. In the USA, the kindergarten year remains optional in some states, and grade school generally begins at 6 as in continental Europe. As Sharp (2002: 15) concludes, 'it is clear that the UK is out of step with other countries in introducing children to school, and thereby to more formal learning, early in life'. Only Northern Ireland and the Netherlands have an earlier starting age, while 15 of the 21 countries surveyed by Bertram and Pascal (2002) have a compulsory start date of 6 years.

Although some UK parents apparently feel that formal learning is beneficial for children, 'the earlier the better', others regret the introduction of such constraints. The important question however may be not 'when do they start?' but 'what do they start?' Full days in the traditional reception classes of the 1960s and 1970s may have been days spent in singing, stories and free play, in and out of doors; whereas full days in the reception classes of the 2000s, despite the mandatory outdoor curriculum, may make far greater demands on young children. It is these demands which may 'dishearten' some children, while for others they are perfectly matched to their inclinations.

Pre-school and school: where does the difference lie?

Most practitioners would confirm from experience the research finding that children who have experience of pre-school provision find the adaptation to school, and school learning, far easier than those who have not. The EPPE study (Sylva et al. 2004) confirms that when 'home' children – those with no experience in a setting before school – start school, they achieve poorer scores for social and emotional development, as well as for academic achievement, than the rest of their cohort, in spite of individual differences in their backgrounds. With the advent of the Foundation Stage for children aged 3 and 4, it might be assumed that children already in nursery, from the age of 3, are offered a smooth bridge into the reception class they enter when they are 4, where the same curriculum and pedagogy is recommended, and familiar buildings and facilities may be shared. There are encouraging signs that this intention is being met in some settings. But there is also a persistent, historically founded, divide between the two environments, in the UK as in most other countries where research has been carried out – a divide based on our conceptions of what a pre-school child, and a school pupil, ought to be *like*.

Researchers such as Anning (1991), Bennett et al. (1997) and Pollard et al. (1994) have identified the fundamental difference between the 'developmental tradition' or 'nursery inheritance' of pre-school education and the 'elementary tradition' of primary education. The two traditions after all have very different roots. Elementary education was conceived from its inception as preparation and training for adult work and adult citizenship; nursery education was conceived as an opportunity for the child's innate potential to grow and blossom. The former contains elements of the factory system (young untrained minds and bodies come in; older, disciplined minds and bodies come out) whereas the latter has echoes of the 'garden' in which children's natural capacities can flourish in their own time.

Neither of these conceptions is inherently inappropriate, but they do incorporate very different images of the child: on the one hand, the 'infant' nurtured by nature and by mother surrogates, on the other hand the 'pupil' disciplined and drilled by expert tutors. The transition between the provision made for these two 'types' of child, these two images of childhood, may be stark. In theory, a child who is viewed at one point in time as a sensitive, developing organism may be classified, only a few weeks later, as a pupil to be disciplined and socialized into conformity and compliance. In practice, teachers in mainstream schooling are humane and sympathetic, and make every effort to treat children as individuals, with different needs. But the system within which they work, with its standards and levels and accountability, may oblige them to focus on meeting targets, rather than on meeting needs and respecting children's right to learn in their own way and at their own pace. These systemic requirements, rather than the actual inclinations of teachers, contribute to the huge gulf that research has identified between children's pre-school experiences and their first experience of school, in the UK and elsewhere.

Pre-school to school: changing expectations

Differences in practitioners' expectations of children in their pre-school and school-pupil incarnations are clearly visible in the research findings from a range of countries. One consistent feature of these is that, perhaps counter-intuitively, pre-school children are generally regarded as more competent and capable by their teachers, than are primary children. To put it simply, pre-school practitioners, on the whole, appear to trust children to make sensible and appropriate choices about their learning and behaviour, while school teachers are less likely to trust children in this way. What follows, inevitably, is that children are often entrusted with greater freedom, and greater responsibility, before they begin formal schooling, than when they reach school age. It may be no surprise therefore if a child who feels *suitable* (Broström 2002) in a nursery classroom feels distinctly *unsuitable* in a primary setting.

A fascinating study (Hendy and Whitebread 2000) of the ways that children aged 3 to 8, and their parents and teachers, understand the idea of 'independent learning', makes this point very clearly in relation to academic progression. These authors used interviews and questionnaires to elicit the views of 48 children from nursery to Year 2. Their findings show that 'independence' is defined very differently by the children, their parents and their teachers. Children, from 3 upwards, wanted to make their own choices and express their own preferences for activities, and were perfectly aware of their own limitations, and of the aspects of learning which required adult help. Their parents endorsed the view that children could think for themselves, and make choices independently, from around the age of 2. The teachers, however, all believed that this independent thinking occurred some time later, and rather surprisingly 'Teachers of the older classes perceive children's independent abilities to be achieved later than their colleagues teaching the younger age groups' (Hendy and Whitebread 2000: 249). When it came to seeking help with difficulties, nursery children (and their teachers) said that children first tried to manage things for themselves, while older children and most adults reported that children would always ask an adult for help first. As the authors report, 'The pattern of responses seems to support the children's view that they become more dependent upon adults, rather than less, during their first few years at school' (Hendy and Whitebread 2000: 251). In consequence, teachers may be fostering a 'dependency culture' which makes children rely increasingly on teachers rather than on their own abilities to learn independently and solve problems as they arise.

So perhaps it is not surprising that a study of children's self-concept at the start of school, and their academic progress during their first year of school (Ramey et al. 1998) concludes that 'in general, young children start school with a high appraisal of their own competencies that declines thereafter' (Ramey et al. 1998: 312). In this study too, the move into formal schooling (American First Grade) was found to offer 'a more structured and demanding school environment in which children's performance is monitored more closely and children's self-control is vital to classroom order' (Ramey et al. 1998: 314). Like the English teachers interviewed by Hendy and Whitebread, the respondents in this study demonstrated that primary-grade teachers work in an environment where the 'independence' children need to demonstrate is the ability to follow instructions and stay on task without constant adult intervention – *not* the kind of independence that nursery teachers are likely to prioritize.

Ramey and colleagues' findings were subsequently confirmed by a nation-wide survey in which 10,000 American teachers were asked about the 'problems' children presented on their first transition to school (Rimm-Kaufman et al. 2000). Amid a complex array of findings, categorized by the social class of the neighbourhood and the ethnicity of the children, comes the stark fact that *half* of those surveyed reported that *half* their class had 'difficulty following directions'. While sympathizing with the teachers, one can only wonder about the experiences of the children who were thus classified, who may not even have realized that 'following directions' was what they were in school for.

What makes school 'disheartening'?

Some children's sense of dismay and disappointment on entering school is conjured up very well by the Plowden committee's choice of word: 'disheartening'. Only a small minority of children are truly upset by separation from parents at this point, and very few are truly fearful of their new environment and teachers. But many may feel a sense of disappointment or anti-climax when the long-awaited 'transition to big school' comes, and many more may feel increasingly discouraged as they learn the rules and routines of the setting which, they come to understand, is where they will spend much of their lives in the weeks, months and years to come.

The word 'disheartening' evokes a striking image: children 'losing heart' as they come to terms with their new experiences. The 'heart' they lose may be a combination of important feelings: enthusiasm, eagerness, confidence, competence or even courage, a rarely used term for normal children in normal circumstances. In *The Wizard of Oz* it is the Tin Woodman who lacks 'heart' but the Cowardly Lion who lacks courage. Children are not cowardly, but they may need to summon up all their reserves of bravery – their ability to proceed with experiences which cause them fear or distress or anxiety – when they make a big transition. Entwisle and Alexander (1998) emphasize the imaginative leap that adults need to make to put themselves in children's shoes, and understand the loss of control over their familiar routines and actions which is experienced by children when they move on from kindergarten:

> The shock of the first grade transition is hard to appreciate. One way for adults to imagine it is to recall their own reactions to being placed in a total institution, for example, how they felt on becoming an inpatient in a hospital, or starting a new job, or going into the army.
>
> (1998: 355).

These authors argue that this particular transition (like the transition to secondary school) occurs at a time when children are frequently experiencing other internal and developmental changes, such that 'the child's external and internal worlds are undergoing profound change *at the same time*' (1998: 352). In consequence, they report, children's enthusiasm for school (their 'heart') drops off steadily: almost all children enjoy kindergarten, but only 62 per cent of first-grade children 'like school a lot', and this figure falls to 29 per cent in sixth grade (1998: 353). The difference, they argue, lies in the ways that society's expectations of children change once they reach the age of statutory schooling:

'elementary schools are socially organized in ways children have not previously experienced, and provide the kind of stimulation society believes is essential for children's development' (1998: 352).

In the UK, Gill Barrett's (1986) work offers many insights into the ways that early 'disheartenment' can quite quickly lead to 'disaffection', as children discover that what they know and think and find important is not necessarily on the agenda of their new teacher. In the early days in school, she found: 'The children were unable to assert what they know, as they frequently did with parents, because there was no expectation that they should, or would, do so. In terms of "knowing" therefore they appeared to be learning that they only knew what the activities and expectations expected of them' (1986: 62).

The children's responses expressed their 'not knowing what to do', identified by Barrett as a major source of distress leading to withdrawal from activities, and also their 'not being involved', leading to apparent tiredness or lack of interest, but possibly masking a fear of failure. The children who 'knew what to do' – those from school-like homes, like Joshua – used the resources they had brought from home to acquire the specialist practical and intellectual skills they needed in the classroom. Those who did not – children like Jelika – were faced with tough challenges to their sense of identity as well as to their feelings of competence.

Ecological transitions: vulnerability and resilience

When she started school, Jelika, despite being a healthy and happy child with a supportive family network, could be classified as especially vulnerable. She was entering an unfamiliar world in which she was unable to communicate through spoken language, unable to identify the expectations of teachers, and unable to guess the meaning of the routines and rituals of the classroom. She made the transition, in Bronfenbrenner's terms, unaccompanied by any experienced person from the known world of her home, who could mediate between the familiar and the strange – no parent, friend, neighbour or sibling, and only rarely a bilingual assistant, when she could be spared from other responsibilities. Her teachers had little information about her background and circumstances, and no means of making strong and supportive links with the family. So in adapting to school, and learning about her new environment, she lacked the scaffolding that supports young children's learning. No one was there who could explain tasks or translate instructions, or identify aspects of an activity and help her to focus on its most important components.

Although Jelika's teachers gave her all the emotional warmth and friendly encouragement they could, the school lacked the structures needed to support children's transitions through the ecological environment. While Joshua's bundle of links between home and school eased his effortless transition into the classroom, Jelika's complete lack of links and support left her to make the transition unaided. The fact that she did so suggests that her resilience, resourcefulness and reciprocity had been acquired during her early years in her family, whose support was invisible to me, but evidently present to her.

These qualities of resilience give children the ability to keep going through 'disheartening' circumstances, and view difficulties and discomforts as challenges to be overcome. Transitional experiences may either dent, or strengthen children's resilience, and all children, especially the 'vulnerable', are entitled to well-planned support to ensure that the outcomes are positive rather than negative. In the next chapter I examine the ways that the transitions of another vulnerable group – babies and toddlers – can be supported, and later chapters will describe other children needing additional provision for their transitions.

Conclusion

This chapter has introduced the range of transitions that young children make in our early 21st-century societies, and some evidence of the impact these transitions may have on them. Changes in demographics, and in our societies' social and working arrangements, have brought about dramatic changes in the ways that young children are cared for and educated in their early years. Though the official 'school-starting age' has remained the same, many children's educational transitions are now much earlier as well as much more frequent. For most children, the 'first transition' is unlikely to be from home to school, or even from home to pre-school.

Nevertheless 'starting school' remains a major event in children's lives, and the head-start afforded by pre-school experiences may not always prepare them for the world of primary school. Children who 'lose heart' at this point will need careful nurturing if they are to recover their resilience before taking the next big step. As Kavkoulis (1994: 42) points out, education is an unending sequence of transitions: 'This progressive stepping and changing in the school levels seems to be a basic structural characteristic of all educational systems'. The task of educators and policy-makers is to understand the impact of these 'steps and changes', and provide the resources children and families require to ensure that the impact is positive.

2

First steps: transitions from birth to 3

Settling in babies: She cried all day, which was heart-breaking. I'd come back and say, 'Did she cry today?' 'Yes'. 'All day?' 'Yes'. She was used to her routine, to breast-feeding, so her whole little life was turned upside down.

(Parent interview, nursery)

Given that life's many transitions can be facilitated, and given how the quality of life's transitions impact our lives, transitions are too important to be left to chance.

(Daniel 1998: 4)

Despite the growing focus on transitions over the last decade, and the wealth of evidence that has flowed from studies around the world, rather little interest has been shown in the first transitions into group care made by babies and toddlers. While increasing numbers of children enter group care when they are a few months old, the focus of research has tended to stay on the more obviously 'educational' transitions into pre-school and school. This chapter uses evidence from a study of children's early experiences of day care in a London children's centre to illustrate the ways that a 'triangle of care' between the child, the parents and the key worker can be constructed by all those involved, as very young children settle in to their new environment.

Early studies of babies' and toddlers' transitions have tended to come from a psychological perspective, and have focused on the role of attachment in children's relationships with their caregivers, and the impact of separation on children's emotional health (Dalli 2000). The important work of Bowlby (1978) and Ainsworth (1978) in describing the ways that bonds are formed between infants and caregivers, and the problems that can arise when these bonds are severed, has tended to overshadow all other approaches to young children's nursery experiences – and may have contributed to the guilt that many mothers describe when their child is first cared for by someone outside the family (Daniel 1998).

Our understanding of attachment, and of the problems of separation, has quite rightly led to a strong focus on 'settling-in' arrangements for babies and toddlers. Most settings have well-developed plans which enable young children to become familiar with their new environment, and form relationships with their new caregivers, at the same time as they gradually become accustomed to their parent's departure and temporary absence. The encouraging message, from the studies that have been undertaken in this field, is that most children appear to be settled and content within a few weeks of starting nursery, even if their first days of separation are distressing (Dalli 1999, 2000). Another strong message, now increasingly taken to heart by policy-makers, is the importance of a 'key person' in the life of the child, and in the nursery of a key worker with whom the child and parents can form a close relationship – a triangle of care. These messages are confirmed by the stories told in this chapter.

I begin the chapter by describing the experiences of three children, aged from 7 months to 25 months, as they settle into their nursery and begin to construct relationships and establish routines within the new environment. Key aspects of their experience are then drawn out and discussed: the ways that relationships are constructed, in a 'caring triangle' (Hohmann 2007) between the child, the parent and the key worker; the contribution of peer friendships to children's well-being and belonging; the importance of routines as a support and scaffold for children; and the sensitive ways that young children's distress over separation can be acknowledged and contained by adults who 'care' for all aspects of the child's identity and well-being. As with older children, the goals for these early transitions can be viewed as fostering the children's well-being, in the present, and endowing them with resilience, resourcefulness and reciprocity as they continue their life-long learning.

The chapter concludes with another case study, of a child whose transition to nursery demonstrates the positive outcomes that can result from thoughtful attention to children's own preferences and those of their parents; and with the lessons of good practice which can be drawn from all such stories.

Starting out in Babies' and Toddlers': three case studies

In September 2006, when this study began, Billy (aged 7 months), Hana (aged 19 months) and Davey (aged 25 months) were all being settled in to their new nursery environments in City Fields Children's Centre: Billy and Hana in the babies' room which catered for children under 2, and Davey in the toddlers' area, which catered for children aged 2 to 3. The nursery has well-established routines for managing transitions – introductions, visits, induction days, home visits, settling-in arrangements – and well-tried strategies to help young children to make a safe and smooth transition. All children are allocated to a key worker who stays close by them in their first few weeks and responds to their needs. But each of the children, for reasons to do with their age, their home experience and their individual preferences, followed a very different path to 'belonging' in the nursery, and the differences in their experiences are as instructive as the similarities.

Billy (7 months)

Billy made a visit to the nursery on Induction Day, and met his key worker, Lillian, who later reported on her first impressions:

> I was in the Parents' Room talking to parents, very much about housekeeping, making sure they've got their start dates and things like that, but he was quite happy to sit there right the way through, so I thought he's a content little baby, he's obviously got a very good relationship with mum and dad ... he was quite happy just sitting there, and he was watching me and watching other people as we were talking.

A week or two later, these impressions were confirmed on the home visit when Lillian picked up further clues:

> He was quite interested with what I brought, because we take a bag of toys and he was quite happy playing with the musical instruments and things like that, so that's something he appeared very keen on, so I thought if I needed anything that would be my key for Billy, that he is interested in sounds and music.

Billy was settled by his dad for the recommended two-week period, but Lillian noted that he appeared relatively independent, and ready to engage with what was offered in the babies' room: 'I did a lot of treasure basket activities, a lot of sensory activities, and he absolutely adored it and he just settled so well ...'. The team discussed his easy transition and agreed that he was probably too young to be vulnerable to real separation anxieties; Billy's range was extended to the outdoor area, where Lillian noted his enjoyment:

> He loves the garden, absolutely loves the garden ... and I think he's very much at the exploring with his senses, putting things in his mouth, watching the leaves fall, he's very much at the awe and wonder stage where everything seems magical!

After four weeks in the setting, Billy had established good relationships with all the adults, and had discovered the pleasure of being with other children. He was happy to be handed over to other staff members when Lillian was not available, and made active efforts to engage with them as well as with the children in his room. Lillian reports:

> I've been doing some observations on Billy, and he does, if he's doing something and a child makes a sound, across the room, he's very much looking to see, and his body language is like that, he wants to go, he's leaning forward, he's just not managing to be mobile yet, but you can see, he's a very sociable child.

This sociability is facilitated by the staff, who recognize that babies and young children enjoy each others' company, and that this is one of the real benefits of being in nursery from an early age. My field notes record:

> Travis wanders into the kitchen area when his mum leaves, and is invited to share some toast with Billy. Jacqui sets up a small table and two chairs so the two little boys can sit face to face and share squares of toast from the same plate; she sits alongside them, chatting, interacting intimately with both of them and drawing them together by focusing on the activity they share, and drawing attention to the way they are sharing their food and their company.

Not long afterwards, Billy finds a new source of interest:

> Still sucking his toast, suddenly he notices Jacqui's nails (which are long, sparkly, and bright orange) and starts to play with them; Jacqui offers her hand and he plays with each finger in

> turn with noisy amusement, pulling at each nail and giggling, separating each finger for a separate attempt

Billy's interests are noted and discussed by all the staff, and these preferences continually inform the care he is offered. One of his principal pleasures, as Lillian has observed, is exploring the phenomenon of a 'big girl', Hana, whose transition has been much less smooth.

Hana (19 months)

Hana has a Danish father and a Greek Cypriot mother, and has travelled all over Europe visiting members of her extended family during her short life. She was away when her home visit was booked, so her 'induction' took place on the first day of the settling-in period. On that day, in Lillian's words, 'she didn't depend on her mum, and mum said she'd been left before and she's very happy, and mum didn't foresee any problems with her'.

This did not prove to be the case once the separation process began. Lillian reported that 'Mum stayed with her for the first few days but was quite keen to go ... but I did say we need to judge this by Hana'. In the event, Hana became increasingly distressed, on parting every morning and periodically throughout the day. Lillian and her colleagues tried a number of strategies for comforting her, and providing her with resources which would reassure her, but many of these strategies required close cooperation with her family, which was not always forthcoming. One of the first problems was with the actual 'goodbyes': the nursery insists that parents always say goodbye to their child, but both Hana's mother and her father sometimes 'snuck out' as the staff described it, denying her the chance to manage her feelings about their departure.

Among the transitional objects the staff find effective are favourite toys from home, and family photos, and both of these were helpful to Hana, so long as her parents remembered them. Lillian reported,

> She started asking for Bear quite a bit, which we asked mum to bring in but unfortunately she kept forgetting, so we ended up having to phone her, and mum would bring it in and leave it at reception, and that seemed to ease her a little bit. We'd phone her up and say she's distressed, could you bring the bear in,

but you'd be going all morning, without the bear, and it just appeared at lunchtime...

There was a long delay too before the family photos were produced, but when they did, Lillian emphasized, 'it was literally just like a magic button!'

She carried them around – she's very close to Dad – she carried his photograph around with her that day, and literally she went to sleep with the photograph in her hand; so what I did, I actually had it scanned so it was always accessible for her ... and from then she seemed to settle in.

Once reconciled to the separation, Hana became one of the most active, engaging and sociable children in the Babies' area. Her relationship with Billy brought pleasure to them both – this observation is very typical:

Hana is passing Billy, who has a basket of sounds objects, and decides to stop and sit down with him; she squats and then kneels a short distance from him, and picks up two metal jar-lids, which she bangs together experimentally; she then repeats the action with more intention and pleasure, and begins to interact teasingly with Billy, who looks at her with interest; she continues to bang, pause, look, tease and turn-take with Billy, and both giggle.

During another observation, Billy reaches out for her from the safety of his cushioned support in the garden, and strokes her hair, while she obediently bows her head to allow him; and it was not uncommon to see the two of them simply grinning and giggling at each other – as Lillian reported, 'he seems to find Hana hysterically funny!'

After five weeks Hana appeared fully settled, and was exploring all the areas, all the activities and all the resources the environment offered her. As Lillian pointed out, she had even begun to 'escape' from the babies' area: 'she also ventures over into Toddlers occasionally which is good, it shows she's not relying on the familiar adults she's got here'.

Davey (25 months)

Davey was allocated a nursery place (in the Toddlers' room) shortly before his second birthday, on the grounds of his father's difficulties in managing his own and his two children's needs. He was very attached to his dad, with whom he spent his whole time while his big brother was in school, and he had to work hard at his transition. His key worker, Sara, made a home visit and played with Davey while a colleague attended to the form-filling: 'I just did a bit of play-partnering with him and it seemed to go quite well … he was quite curious about what was in the bag, he showed me things, he was quite excitable'.

Davey's father spent a long time at the nursery settling him in, with active support from Sara:

> When dad was around he'd sort of look out for him but he'd go off and play, and if he was on the truck outside he would check that dad was still there, and then what I used to separate him, when he was just going for the first half hour – we keep it to a short period of time – I'd say daddy's just going to pop to the toilet, so dad went away for maybe 20 minutes, and then we'd keep to that, so, build up reassurance during the day, dad's gone for a cup of tea, or dad's coming back after dinner …

Davey was calm and solemn in this period, and rather wary. For several weeks Sara remained alert to moments when he was apt to become distressed, and used her observation of his interests and temperament to inform her own strategies, both for supporting Davey's separation from his dad, and helping him to cope with the long nursery day:

> I was using things I would do in the mornings, we were using feeding the fish as a distraction: he didn't want to let go but I would say, 'daddy's coming back – shall we go and feed the fish?' That was the thing that I used for quite a few days and he really enjoyed that … and then the following week he just said goodbye to dad.

Like many children in the nursery Davey was helped by understanding the pattern of the day – outdoors, snack, lunch, sleep, play, tea, then daddy! Sara explains:

> He got the routine established and I would talk him through that during the day, so he asked me frequently. There are quite

a few children that we have that frequently ask about the routines of the day and Davey needs that for security.

After six weeks, Sara described Davey as 'looking very settled in the environment', and reported with some surprise that he had begun to be more overtly affectionate in his relationship with her:

Davey is not a very tactile child whereas other children are, they want to be on your lap. Davey doesn't come for that kind of attention, but just recently he has started to, he just runs up, puts his arm round my legs, and then just runs off again.

Davey's dad confirmed that Davey 'just took to Sara straight away, it's the way she puts herself across to him', and that now he was settled he would 'run up and say hello through the window' as he arrived in the morning. Davey had not yet formed any attachments to other children, but the world of the nursery was his, and he looked as if he felt at home there.

First steps: constructing the triangle of care

Billy, Hana and Davey all made a successful first transition, but each of them settled in a different way, supported by an adult who followed the child's own lead, and to a greater or lesser extent by parents who worked with the staff for the benefit of the child. Key aspects of the caring triangle constructed around each of them are considered next.

The notion of 'care', especially 'childcare', has received a great deal of attention in the last few years (Brannen and Moss 2003). One reason for this has been the ongoing debate over the 'care' and 'education' aspects of early childhood services: most practitioners working with young children reject the distinction between the two functions, and argue that everyone who cares for children is an educator, and all educators are care givers. Another reason has been the challenge mounted to traditional ideas of 'care', as something done *for* somebody (a less capable person) *by* somebody else (a more capable person). In many instances, the person who is cared for is a child, and the person who does the caring is a woman, but this need not be the case of course. Theorists have drawn attention to the many different aspects of caring, such as 'caring about', 'taking care of', 'care giving' and 'receiving care', and have argued that the relationship is more than simply one way, and that it involves *feeling* as well as *doing* (Tronto 1993; Sevenhuijsen 1998). In the case of young children in nurseries, it is likely that the care relationship is defined far more by the bonds of affection between the child and care giver, than by the nappy-changing and face-wiping aspects of the job (the physical care).

The caring triangle: key workers and parents

Looking after babies and toddlers is emotional labour, for both parents and professionals, and recognition of this important component of care helps to construct the triangle of care which links the child, the parent and the worker. A young child's entry into a setting often has a huge impact on her parents: as Lillian, the key worker described earlier, reported, 'I see my job, especially in the baby room, more as settling, or as much settling the parents in, as you are settling the children in'. The relationship between key worker and parents is a key component of the settling-in process. It is the time when the 'expert' knowledge of the parent (of her own child) meets the 'expert' knowledge of the practitioner (of children in general), and when both must learn to trust and respect each other.

Many aspects of the child's transition depend on how this relationship goes. As Hohmann (2007: 33) warns (from a study of childminders): 'a combination of expectations from parents and practitioners regarding everyday care practice can either be the basis of a trusting relationship between the adults involved in this caring triangle or a breeding-ground for tension'. At City Fields Children's Centre, both staff and parents acknowledge the importance of the link between them: a key worker commented on settling a new child that 'for me it was my relationship with mum that I had to really think about'.

Where parents are already known to staff through the attendance of older siblings, as in 2-year-old Jack's case, there is a huge advantage. Sara, his key worker explains:

> I had a good relationship with mum, and I saw Jack – well, talked to mum when she was pregnant and saw him when he was born, so we were quite familiar ... as mum and I know each other well and we just sat together chatting, there's quite a difference because mum is so used to the room, and we're having a very comfortable chat, and I think children pick on that, how their parents are feeling ... so some children have that advantage, their mum doesn't need settling!
>
> (Key Worker Interview, Toddlers)

Jack's mother made similar comments on the relationship:

It's quite informal actually although she's his key worker; I tell her how he's doing, or how I think he's doing, and stuff that's going on at home, and we have a chat and a laugh, it's quite relaxed ... I think the personal relationship is very important in nursery, in this age group, the fact that you have that kind of atmosphere, because of the trust, because they are so little.

Parents understand how important this relationship is. A father whose child had 'moved up' from Toddlers to the over-3s area emphasized that 'it's a real bond, an emotional one, because you're forever grateful that this person's taken care of your child'. Hana's mother further explains:

Lillian made me very comfortable, she made me feel, your child is safe here, we do this and this, trying to explain things they're doing every day, so obviously when you come back and children are happy, you start to trust them.

(Parent Interview, Babies)

It is understood by both parents and staff that there is a real overlap of their roles and relationships with the child – that both provide extremely intimate, and affectionate, care for the child – but that the relationship between them as adults remains a professional one: key workers may go off duty, or give up their job, but parents rarely do so!

The caring triangle: key workers and children

The relationship between the key worker and the child is the most critical aspect of small children's transitions. Although the adult may initially appear to take the lead in establishing a relationship, it is clear from the different forms this relationship takes that children actively shape the process during their settling-in period, and that over time they co-construct with their key worker the type of bond that suits their own needs and preferences. For some children, the initial relationship may be one of close attachment and dependence, which is gradually eased and relaxed as the child gains confidence. For others there may be an initial determination to maintain some independence and detachment from their new care giver, which similarly becomes less imperative as the child develops trust. Dalli (2000) argues that children's relationships with adults in childcare settings are shaped by the particular expectations of the setting, which the child is required to work with and negotiate. But at City Fields, it appeared that the golden rule of always 'following the child', or 'going by the child', meant that each child was free to set the rules of the relationship for themselves.

None of the key workers at City Fields felt that their own relationship with their key children in any way resembled a parent's, although they acknowledged that their own roles – feeding, changing, comforting, playing, getting to sleep – were often essentially similar to those of parents. Although they acknowledged the intimacy of the tasks they undertook with the child, and even referred to the fact that the child might spend more of her waking hours in their care than in parental care, they still felt that there were significant differences in the relationships they formed. Part of the 'emotional labour' for practitioners involves maintaining these boundaries in their role, and observing the 'feeling rules' which enable a professional care giver to stay a little detached from their key children (see Buchbinder et al. 2006):

> We are definitely not a parent: they are there for them 24 hours a day but we are just providing a service … They see us as a friend, as educators, as another human being who is helping them and who they can play with.
>
> (Key Worker, Kindergarten)

This particular (male) key worker expresses, like many of his colleagues, what we might call the 'view from the child': key workers' responsibility is to be available when the child needs a playmate, a comforter, a helpmeet or an emotional support, rather than to be either a constant presence, or someone who can demand reciprocal attention:

> He just comes to me for comfort, if he gets upset; and sometimes if he's coming in from the garden he'll just call my name and just check that I'm there, so I suppose it's just that bit of security…
>
> (Key Worker, Toddlers)

Lillian, although she cares for some of the youngest children in the centre, is equally sure that her role is not that of a parent: 'I think if you had to put a name to it I would say it's just like having a best friend. Somebody that you can go to, somebody that you know is always going to be there for you'.

All the key workers interviewed for this study explained that the nature of the relationship was shaped by the child's own wishes; that some children wish for more explicit and visible shows of affection, and attention, whereas others prefer to maintain their independence as far as possible. In this respect it is clear that the adults' professional role requires them to make fewer demands of the children themselves than a parent might, although several admitted how hard it could be to say goodbye to children when it was time for their next transition.

Beyond the caring triangle

At the same time as children are supported in constructing the relationships that suit their needs, within the intimacy of the triangle of care, they are also being inducted into the much wider social worlds of the group, and the nursery as a whole. Key workers have to develop strategies for supporting children through all the new challenges that this entry into the wider world brings with it. I describe here some of the important factors that foster children's well-being as members of a larger group than they have previously experienced: understanding routines, enjoying relationships, and identifying the links between their two separate worlds.

Understanding routines

Learning the routines of the nursery day is an important step towards feeling in control, and feeling a sense of belonging, in the new environment. For the youngest children, however, it was the staff's ability to mirror the routines of home that was the first priority. During the home visit, key workers see for themselves, and inquire about, the routines which make up the young child's daily life. For babies and toddlers, these may focus to a large extent on being comforted when upset or sleepy. Sara gives an example:

> We ask a lot about how does, which part of the day does the child enjoy most, how do they feel when they wake up, generally, what's their routine for going to sleep, and for Jack it's stroking your arm, that's what he likes to do before going to sleep, and he'll do that to me during lunchtime as well, when he's beginning to get tired, he'll just kind of nuzzle in and start stroking because he's getting tired and he's just wanting a comfort – so that was one of the things mum said to me, he likes to stroke your arm to go to sleep, so I was aware of that and he did it pretty much straight away.
> (Key Worker interview, Toddlers)

Comforting, feeding, sleeping and nappy changing recur throughout the day in the babies' room, and if well managed they contribute to the calm and contented atmosphere. Lillian explains that 'we just try to go by the child: that's the key, especially when you're working with babies'.

At the same time, most children quickly learn that the nursery has its own routines, which the key workers use very consciously to induct the child into a sense of belonging. Even small children, who are unable to respond to 'clock time', seem to understand the sequence of the day when it is narrated to them by their nursery workers, as Sara explains:

> I think some of them are able to work out the time scale ... we've got older toddlers who can go through the routines for themselves but I think Jack is – I don't talk to him too much about the routine because I think too much information, but just a little bit of information about what's happening, lunch, sleep, play and then mummy's coming back, she's going to pick up Martin and then she'll be here.
>
> (Key Worker Interview, Toddlers)

Even in the babies' room, some children were observed to have a good grasp of these routines and to follow cues for the day's main events with considerable confidence. Lillian offered the example of Liam, aged 16 months:

> He knows the routine; we'll go in and it'll be lunchtime and he'll go straight to the bathroom because he knows we have to wash our hands before lunch; or I'll say we're going in the garden and he'll immediately go and get his coat, things like that.

As she explained, 'I think there are routines that are predictable, things like lunchtime and stuff like that, they are predictable, but then again we do talk to the children an awful lot about routines!'. Talking about routines supports children's growing individual ability to take control of their day, but also helps to bond the children together in a social group with shared experiences, a small community of early learners.

Enjoying relationships

As the case studies of Hana and Billy suggested, the company of other children contributes enormously to young children's pleasure in their new surroundings. The sociability of babies, which parents and practitioners have always noticed, is clearly demonstrated by research (Goldschmied and Jackson 1994; Murray and Andrews 2000) and few would now argue that children under 3 are 'too young to make friends' (Dunn 2004). Thyssen (2000: 39) offers some lovely examples of the affectionate initiatives of a 12-month old girl settling in to a Danish nursery:

> Sarah reaches out and Tom puts his head forward, as if he wants to be stroked or to kiss her. 'Ha ha ha' Sarah says happily.
>
> [first day in day care]

Sarah crawls up to John. At first she sits looking at him for a bit, then she pats him cautiously on the hair. She hums tenderly.

[Two weeks in day care]

A boy comes up to Sarah and reaches out. 'Doi, dori, doi' Sarah says happily and reaches out towards him.

[Four weeks in day care]

Thyssen's observations confirm that pleasurable interactions of this kind, which constitute age-appropriate friendships for very young children, support them in separating from home care givers. But like older children they may require support for their friendships, and a structure which brings them together in activities where they can become aware of each other, and of the rewards of shared experiences. In the Danish day care settings, staff did not seem concerned to facilitate these encounters, which the children managed on their own initiative, often using objects as a form of self-presentation or introduction (Thyssen, 2000).

At City Fields, one of the key worker's roles is to foster attachments between children, rather than simply to foster children's attachments to their key worker. It is in this sense that the key workers often describe themselves as 'like a friend' to their key children. A friend, they say, is someone who is 'there when you want them', 'helps them to fit in', and 'plays when they need someone to play with'. They can offer affection and comfort that is different from a parent's, while helping the child to understand that it is possible to manage their day away from a parent. A key worker explains:

I'd like to think I'm their friend. I use this quite a lot, if they're upset, I say, 'would you like a little cuddle? I know my cuddle's not as good as mummy's cuddle but I can give you my cuddle now and then we'll wait and mummy will come and she'll give you a nice big cuddle'.

(Key Worker Interview, Toddlers)

'Friends' are also willing to play what you want to play, and in this respect the key workers at City Fields, as a consequence of their close observations of children, make extremely good friends, who plan opportunities for each child based on their observed preferences and on information from parents.

They plan equally carefully for the small group of children to whom each child becomes attached as part of their transition. 'Key groups' of three or four children meet together with their key worker for a 'special time' in a 'special place' at the start of each day. The special place is a corner of the room decorated with photographs of the children and their families and friends, where the group comes together for a period of intimate chat and sharing. This particular 'routine' is soon learned, and observations show even pre-verbal children's eager and intense body language as they participate in listening to a song quietly sung to them, or a picture book or photograph placed in their hands.

> Sara's key group time: the three children sit close together on their sofa, with Sara in a chair in front. They choose who to 'say hello' to first and each child is softly sung to and engaged individually, examining their clothes, socks, face, feelings, cuts and scratches, and tales from home ('dad cut my hair!'); each child is asked who brought them to nursery, and what happened on the way; then what they would like to do, and where: Jack and Davey both plan to be Batman, in the garden.
>
> (Field notes, Toddlers)

As Sara explains, 'that 15 minutes when they just get to sit with you is really important ... and it's those little things – what socks they're wearing, which adults may think are not very important, but they just love telling you, what they've got on today'.

Almost all the parents who were interviewed, including Billy's and Hana's, named the company of other children when they were asked, 'what they like best' about being in nursery. In the opinion of Billy's mum, 'having the other children there is a big thing for him, although he can't move around ... he does enjoy having them around him'. In turn, Hana's mum describes the aspect of this relationship which has helped Hana – 'caring' for smaller children like Billy:

> With the younger children around her she can show affection, she brought a dolly with her but she can show her emotions with the younger ones and that is why I think children need other children around them, they are more comfortable ...

The evidence from City Fields, including the following example, suggests that the sociability of babies and toddlers contributes to making their daily experience in group care settings highly pleasurable.

Making links with the world outside

From their earliest days in the centre, children are supported in understanding that there are different domains in their lives, and that the world outside the nursery continues to exist while they are not a part of it: there is no attempt to make children 'forget' about their home and family while they are in the centre, or to distract them from their temporary unhappiness over losing them. Children are frequently reminded by their key workers that their mothers will be on their way to work, or picking up an older sibling from school, and encouraged to understand the links between the nursery and the 'outside world'. One morning routine demonstrated this strategy very clearly: although the children were too young to participate in the conversation, they were treated as full participants.

> Lillian sits on cushions at the foot of the floor-length window which looks out on to the entrance courtyard, encouraging the three boys to look out and engage with the outside world. With her help they greet mothers arriving at the centre, and discuss who they are ('there's Ava's mummy, do you think that's Ava in the buggy?'), and look out for the same mothers leaving after depositing children. Then they look out for staff arriving ('Jacqui should be here soon: which way do you think she'll come?'); they greet and discuss the cook, the caretaker, and their work; they wave hello and goodbye to everyone including departing mums.
>
> (Field notes, Babies Room)

The key groups described earlier are also opportunities for staff to focus on the links with home, asking children to recall who dressed them and brought them to nursery, and where that adult was going to be during the day. Most parents supply family photos at the staff's request, and these are displayed and discussed as part of the daily routine, but the child's life in the nursery is also celebrated, as another key worker reports:

> The children took photographs of one another ... so I incorporated that into their special place; so we made the backing for the wall, we took photos and then I took photos of them playing together, so they had that sense of belonging at nursery, and then they had their photos from home which was their sense of belonging at home, and we put them together, and the children then started to name each other and one another's families, and I think that really helped me with the children, we'd say, 'who's this one, who's this climbing over that, oh that's Shabna' and that's the way it went on and I think it really helped them to settle.
>
> (Key Worker interview, Toddlers)

Links in the mesosystem

Observing the youngest children make the transition into City Fields showed once again the value of Bronfenbrenner's analysis of what makes a 'good' transition – good for the child and family in the immediate moment, and good for the child's longer-term development. As he argued, it seems clear that, the more links there are between the microsystems of home and nursery, and the stronger these links are, the better the child's transition experience is likely to be.

The triangle of care that supports each child offers a sustaining network of links at the face-to-face level, through the experience of home visits by the key worker, and nursery visits by the family, as well as through daily conversations. It needs to include high levels of trust and respect between parents and practitioners: in Hana's case this trust was slightly jeopardized by her parents' unwillingness to follow the nursery's advice in the settling-in period, whereas other parents made every possible effort to communicate their own knowledge about their child, and to take advantage of the key workers' knowledge of 'children'. At the children's own level, it is supported by the presence in the nursery of photographs of home and nursery, family and friends, side by side; and by the transitional objects such as blankets or soft toys which the child may bring for security, even if she never needs them and they stay on the shelf.

For children under 3, for whom the experience of 'transition' from one microsystem to another occurs every day, the supportive links need to be continually renewed. The final case study in this chapter illustrates a trusting relationship between home and setting.

Case study: Yuk-Yue (26 months)

Yuk-Yue made the transition to the Toddlers' area in September, along with Davey. She was a self-possessed and competent child, the youngest of five siblings in a Chinese family, and did not appear to need specific support from adults in her early days in nursery. Rather than attaching herself to Kerry, her key worker, and then gradually letting go, she initially chose independence, and then in her own time came to construct a closer relationship. Kerry summed this up:

> She takes a while getting to know an adult and I'm still getting to know her ... she's always known she can come to me and get help but I think our relationship is stronger in the last

couple of weeks than it has been since she started, and that real relationship has taken me a while with her. Now, over the last couple of weeks, she comes in and shows me things she's brought from home. So she did a lot of the settling, I've got to say that …

The closer relationship established from her fourth week in the nursery was the result of initiatives by both child and adult, and on Kerry's part was based on observing Yuk-Yue at home and in the home corner in the nursery:

It started with a cooking activity with her, because I decided to do a week of cooking activity, to try and support that interest in the home corner, and it really worked, not just for her, it worked for other children's needs as well, and it created that bond with her.

The shared activity also helped to integrate Yuk-Yue into her key group:

With Yuk-Yue, she's a very physical child, she can be here, she can be there, she can be climbing, so she's rushing around so I think that was why she sometimes didn't have that time to bond with everyone, so the cooking activity, they were sitting together, and they needed to pass things to one another, and that brought her in with the group and that tied her in with me as well.

Observations confirmed that Yuk-Yue was identifiably 'tied in' with adults, children, activities and the environment by her fifth week in the nursery. While being observed she made confident overtures to a range of individuals:

She has been talking to Clair, who now leaves the conservatory to go in the garden; another key worker comes by and Yuk-Yue climbs on to her lap and hugs her with a big squeeze. They chat briefly then this key worker also passes on into the garden.

(Field notes, week 4)

She is playing in the sand indoors alongside other children; she approaches a new staff member as she enters the room and gives her a tin of sand with a spoon in it (and is thanked). Then goes to collect a new container of sand which she takes to Kerry (sitting at the malleable activity); Kerry enacts pleasure and gratitude and offers this 'drink' to the children sitting with her.

(Field notes, week 5)

Kerry described how cautious she had been in her approach to Yuk-Yue, watching for signs of the way she liked to be cared for and waiting for her to demonstrate her preferences. As she emphasized, 'some children would be mortified if you picked them up and cuddled them, some children like it, you have to take that into consideration, because if you go in and just swoop up a child, that doesn't want to be comforted or doesn't know you well enough for a cuddle ...'. With Yuk-Yue, physical closeness developed over time:

> Now if you go up to her and touch her – a little rub on her cheek or a little tickle, it really brings a smile to her face, she's got this smile, so that's a really big thing that's moved on and she'll often come and lean against my leg, or she'll bring a chair to sit beside me, and the conversation is starting to build as well.

Yuk-Yue's mother's confidence in Kerry made the caring triangle complete:

> Sometimes I'm in a rush in the morning and Yuk-Yue will feel that insecurity and will say – I don't like you go! – and then I say, 'Yuk-Yue, say Bye Bye Mummy' and Kerry will be holding her and say, 'Shall we say goodbye to mummy? Through the window?' That is a professional skill, to calm children through the professional way. They are very strict about this rule, I tell the child I am going and I am coming back.

Interestingly, both mum and Kerry answered the question, 'how can you tell that she feels she belongs here?' by describing Yuk-Yue's arrival at the setting every morning: her sense of belonging is shared by key worker and parent.

> You can tell when children come with a smile – some children need to be brought in, they'll stand outside the classroom; other children just come in on their own and I think if they cross that door on their own, without an adult, to me that's when they're starting to feel like, this is *my* area, this is me, this is where I'm happy; I belong here – I don't need an invitation, I

can just come in and be here and play with what I want to, it's
ownership … and Yuk-Yue comes in with a smile!
(Key Worker interview)

When she arrives! Oh yes, because she stands here, she sings a
song and runs on in!
(Parent Interview)

Lessons of good practice for babies and toddlers

Many of the practices observed at City Fields are replicated in other
nurseries. Home visits by the key worker, extended settling-in periods,
and the very gradual withdrawal of parental support for the child, are
standard practice in good nurseries, where most small children make
successful transitions and can be seen to demonstrate a sense of
belonging, within weeks of the move.

While arrangements like these should be written into every nursery's
policy, other aspects of good practice are harder to prescribe, and rely on
the overall ethos (and the good leadership) which permeates the setting.
Some of these could be described as follows:

- A key worker system which allows a new child to be offered close
  and constant support in her early days in the setting – at City Fields
  additional staff are made available so that the new child has unin-
  terrupted care – and also enables parents to receive all the
  information and reassurance they need at this time.
- A respect for the individuality of each child, which implies that a new
  child's preferences must be inferred both through discussion with
  parents and through careful monitoring of the child's responses (to
  physical contact, tone of voice, changes in routine and so on).
- Close attention to building a relationship with each child's parents, so
  that the triangle of care is completed through friendly and trusting
  exchanges which allow differences of approach to be resolved before
  they can result in tensions or disagreements which will impact on the
  child.
- Support for the child's peer relationships, including well-planned
  strategies for including even the youngest children in group activities
  (rather than assuming that they are at the stage of 'solitary play').
- Support for child-friendly daily routines which are predictable
  enough to offer the young child security and a sense of control, but
  flexible enough to allow for individual differences in activity patterns, and different expectations brought from home.

- Constant and explicit links made between home and setting: through photos, objects and activities, but also through *talking* about home, family and the journey to school, and about the expected return of mum or dad.

Conclusion: *acquiring the* 3 Rs *(or* 4)

Although parents may anticipate their child's transition with some anxiety, we know that most young children do settle well, with the support of sensitive care givers. We know too that a positive experience of early transition will strengthen their '3 Rs' and help them to approach subsequent transitions equally positively. Experiencing life in two domains, and developing new forms of identity, supports children's *resilience*, so long as those domains and identities are carefully and constructively linked; experiencing new activities and environments enhances *resourcefulness*, giving a child more knowledge, skills and information to draw on in the future; and making new relationships within a happy, sociable setting encourages *reciprocity*, the belief that sharing and collaborating brings positive outcomes. As with all transitions, a final factor to be considered is the child's 'readiness' – a positive disposition towards new experiences, new environments and new relationships. The City Fields children show definite signs of taking their first steps in this direction.

3

Bridging cultures: home, pre-school and school

Leaving home and going to pre-school for the first time was exciting for me. I went with my mother because I did not know anybody. My first day was strange. I told my mother to stay with me until lunch so we can go back home together. Then after three days I made friends. I told my mother not to come with me to pre-school because I can come alone.

(Pre-school child, Fiji)

If the culture of the teacher is to become part of the consciousness of the child, then the culture of the child must first be in the consciousness of the teacher.

(Bernstein 1970: 31)

The last chapter has shown the good outcomes that are evident when small children have the opportunity to receive close individual attention during their transition into a new setting: when they are cared for by adults who watch and wait, follow their preferences and support their development through careful planning. The key workers explained that their practice was based on recognizing the *individuality* of each child, and the children flourished in response.

As they go through the school system, children inevitably come to be seen, not just as individuals, but also as 'types' of children: just as adults do, they acquire labels which shape the ways we interact with them and the expectations we hold for them. We think of them, not just as 'that individual child' but also as 'one of the shyer Bengali children' or 'one of the more boisterous boys'. Any child starting school or pre-school belongs to one or more of these types, and just as all children need their schemas to make sense of the world, so all practitioners need to call on these types to help them to make sense of individual children and plan for their needs. The most obvious categories of course include gender (do girls settle better than boys?) and age (do 2-year-olds settle more quickly than 1-year-olds?) but the myriad other categories into which we, largely unconsciously, sort children, include children with special needs and other forms of vulnerability, and children from different social class or ethnic backgrounds.

We need to understand the different 'cultures' of children's backgrounds in order to understand the nature of the transitions that they make when they start in pre-school settings at the age of 3 or 4. Children of this age are generally cared for in larger groups, with larger ratios, than under-3s, and are less likely to have exclusive access to a key worker as they settle in. So the intimate knowledge of the child's home experience and routines which helps settings to mirror an infant's home experience is less likely to inform the transitions of older children, despite the best efforts of the school or pre-school. For this reason we tend to call on our own 'common-sense knowledge', or sometimes on research knowledge, about the characteristics of different families and communities. The problem is, of course, that such 'types' can easily turn into stereotypes, which hide rather than reveal the characteristics of a particular family's environment and practices.

This chapter explores the idea of 'culture' more generally, arguing that every family has its own unique home culture, which shares some characteristics with similar families but is the product of beliefs and values which the family members have acquired through their own life-experiences. The theoretical ideas of the French sociologist Pierre Bourdieu are introduced as a means to clarify and illuminate the ways that such home cultures – he uses the term *habitus* – develop, and what happens when children bring their home *habitus* to school. The examples of two girls, both starting their educational journey in Foundation Stage settings in England, are used to illustrate the ways that 'home' beliefs, practices and expectations can shape children's dispositions towards their new settings, making their transition more or less comfortable. A key focus of these beliefs, once again, is the idea of 'readiness', since this concept informs the ways that parents prepare their children for school, and the ways that practitioners respond to the young children in their care. The chapter concludes by summarizing the barriers which can grow up between children's familiar world and the unfamiliar world of school; and the bridges which can be built to ensure them a safe passage across to their new world.

Bridging cultures: Saskia and Sonia

Saskia, aged 3, and Sonia, aged 4, joined their respective nursery and reception classes in different settings and different cities. Both girls grew up in caring and supportive English families, and both entered welcoming early years' environments, but the relationship that developed between the familiar world of home, and the unfamiliar new setting, was very different for each of them. Their circumstances, though unique to each child, derive from aspects of the family culture in which each has been raised.

Saskia (aged 3)

Saskia is the only child of professional parents who work flexible hours, and have no difficulty in making time for settling-in routines, or for dropping by the nursery for chats. Saskia's earliest experiences of group care were with a childminder, where she was very happy. As her dad, Matt, reported, 'she settled well – obviously we made a very careful choice, spent some time looking, found someone we were sure was the right person'. When it came to starting nursery, her parents were rather concerned because they had planned a lengthy absence in the States, with relatives, at the time the settling-in was planned. The nursery however 'was flexible, they seem to have the capacity to kind of work around that' and the short series of visits Saskia undertook on her return proved to be sufficient for her to settle and 'stay all day' very rapidly.

Much of the 'settling', it was clear, took place in the family, where Saskia was helped to understand that her future transitions would be positive and pleasurable. Matt explained,

> I think it's really important, helping children through this transition in life, to give them this sense of where they are in the process, it's a kind of hierarchy but a fun hierarchy, from being a baby in the childminder's ... we talked about that, and all along she understood she was on a kind of journey, and it was healthy and natural, and nothing kind of traumatic about it, and there were different stages in life ...

When Saskia met Asima, her key worker, he added, the family had the sense that she was 'going from one set of arms to another'. They encouraged Saskia to understand that 'there's no shortage: when you meet somebody else nice in your life you don't lose the person left behind. So, she's spent a lot of time with other people, but then *we* don't disappear!' This positive preparation was reinforced by Saskia's discovery that some of her old friends from the childminder's were already at the nursery, and that other children from the neighbourhood would soon be starting.

In Saskia's first visits, Asima found her rather reserved: 'initially she came across as quite a shy person who stayed quite close to me'. The organization of the day in this nursery can seem quite complex (key groups, focus groups, language groups, maths groups) and Asima remarked that children can take some time to figure out that 'if this is the language group it's not the same children as the key group – so there's a lot to learn, and a lot to get used to, just being here'. She observed Saskia closely, and played alongside her, for her first few days, and helped her to become involved with a group of friends ('the girl power group' as Matt described it). Once this was established, she explained, 'they can go away a bit more but they know I'm the person they can come back to'. By her fourth week in nursery, observations showed Saskia involved in complicated play planning and negotiations with a group of girls, throughout a whole morning in the garden.

Saskia's home visit had enabled Asima to learn more about her, and the family photos she brought in helped to make her home experience a part of her nursery experience. But her parents in turn made an effort to learn about the nursery's routines and to build them into their family life. Her dad reported that, 'it's part of our kind of family myth, almost, that we all sing the "hello" song – you know, "hello, hello, hello, it's nice to be with you", all that stuff, we have a little singsong sometimes and that's embedded in the kind of family story really'.

Saskia's transition was a thoroughly well-supported, well-planned, family affair, and the arrangements made for her met Bronfenbrenner's 'hypotheses' in all respects. The close relationship which quickly developed between her family and the nursery staff was based on a great sense of trust and optimism on the part of her parents, and rather unusually they had been explicit in communicating their own feelings to Saskia. The parents' confidence in the nursery stemmed in part from a confidence in their own judgement, and their ability to make good choices – as they had in choosing a childminder – and from their sense of their own competence in their dealings with other professionals and with the education system.

Sonia (aged 4)

Sonia started in Reception as one of the oldest in her year group, alongside children who were only just 4 while she was nearly 5. She also started as one of twins: her brother Robbie was her companion and shadow from the first induction visit, and the first day of school.

The twins lived with their mum and four older siblings in a house close to the school, but the family were not really integrated into the neighbourhood. Their mum, Kath, had had a difficult adolescence herself, and been excluded from school before she became pregnant at 15. She remained close to her own parents, who were doting grandparents for the twins, but avoided close contact with other families, and seemed to be wary of professionals of every description. She was, however, absolutely dedicated to the twins' well-being and achievement, and directed a lot of her time to supporting their education at home.

Kath had her own understanding of 'readiness' and the prerequisites for starting school, and as a result had taught the children letters, numbers and colours from an early age, and read them stories from a small collection acquired as the older siblings went through school:

> I did all that with them, I have tried. They should know some letters, we've looked at little dictionaries and different letters, Sonia more than Robbie ... I read them a story and make them copy a sentence out of a book – again, she's more keen than him.

At Kath's request, the twins' older siblings also sometimes 'did sums' and 'tested them'. She had twice attempted to enrol the twins in local pre-schools, but both times, she reported 'they were never happy there so I kept them home a lot'.

When the twins started school they displayed all of their mum's reticence and wariness. Their teacher and nursery nurse welcomed the family warmly, but Kath did not find it easy to overcome her reserve, and stood to one side of the classroom saying very little. After she left each morning, Sonia responded, whispering, to the adults' overtures, and wandered slowly round the room, inspecting the activities with some interest but refusing invitations to try them (Robbie simply stayed silent, and stared). But as time went on, and Robbie began to get involved in solitary play of his own choosing, Sonia continued to remain for long periods alongside an activity but not engaged with it: my field notes described her as 'watching other children at a distance', 'closely examining her own socks and shoes', or trying unsuccessfully to catch Robbie's eye.

After some weeks Sonia, like Saskia, joined a group of girls and began to come out of her shell socially. She silently complied with most adult invitations to join activities, and participated appropriately in learning tasks, although always with one eye on Robbie or on other groups in the room. Her mum spoke appreciatively of the efforts made by the teachers, and of the twins' progress, but reported that she felt her children were 'not learning as much as we did when I went to school'. Nevertheless, she concluded, 'the school does its best – and evidently they quite like it'.

Sonia was supported, in the way they knew best, by her family and her teachers, but there were few links between the two, and none that could help Sonia to make sense of her two worlds. Kath's own experiences had not encouraged her to feel confident about her ability to shape her own life, or to act as an advocate for her children in the school. Although she made determined efforts on behalf of the twins, her ideas of school readiness – learning letters and numbers – did not match those of the staff, who looked for confidence and communicative skills in children. Unlike Saskia, Sonia had not learned to feel trust in the new people she met, or optimism in the new situations she encountered.

Culture: an environment for growing up in

A great deal has been talked and written about 'culture'. It is a word we use daily: to describe the customs and practices of different 'cultural groups'; or to describe the different behaviours of children coming to us from 'culturally diverse' families. It is a word described by Raymond Williams (1976: 76), the great cultural critic, as 'one of the two or three most complicated words in the English language', because it has undergone so many transformations in its long history. But for our present purposes it may be helpful to go back to its earliest meaning, defined by Williams as 'a noun of process: the tending of something, basically crops or animals' (1976: 77); or, by extension to human cultures, the tending of babies and young children.

When human families or communities wish to tend something – whether lambs, tomato plants or human toddlers – they create, to the best of their abilities, the environment that they believe will accomplish their aims of nurturing these young organisms, keeping them alive, and helping them to develop towards maturity. (It is no coincidence that in the English language 'nurseries' are places for the care and nurture of plants, as well as children). As Cole (1998: 15) explains, 'From earliest times, the notion of culture included a general theory for how to promote development: create an artificial environment in which young organisms could be provided optimal conditions for growth'.

The environments created by families are not 'artificial' in the sense that they are fake, simply in the sense that they are 'fashioned' for a particular purpose: we protect babies, as we do seedlings, from frost and drought; we offer warmth and comfort while they are small and vulnerable, and special kinds of food and stimulation as they grow and develop. Some aspects of this cultural childrearing are widely shared, and possibly even universal among human families. Others are very culture-specific: in some countries, parents put children to sleep in silent, darkened rooms away from the rest of the family, while in others, children are expected to sleep and wake on the laps and backs of adults and older children, surrounded by noise and activity. Similar contrasts have been found in all aspects of childrearing: in the ways that adults speak to young children (where the speech we call 'motherese' is not as universal as we once supposed), and in the types of close relationships that are formed (where the mother–child dyad of western cultures does not suit the typical conditions of the majority world) (Harkness 1980; Schieffelin and Ochs 1986).

When children make their first transitions out of the family and into other forms of care, the 'artificial environments' become increasingly specialized. Nurseries and pre-schools reflect the typical beliefs of their local culture about the best ways to care for children, and the most effective ways to educate them. Many of these beliefs are visible in the physical environment, where light and airy spaces, bright colours, natural materials and well-designed resources are generally understood to promote children's happiness, well-being and development. Other beliefs are enshrined in the routines of the day, which are designed to ensure that children's physical, social and emotional needs are met. Practitioners, as we have seen, make conscientious efforts to mirror the routines of young children's home lives, and to offer similar care and comfort.

Other aspects of home cultures are less visible, and harder to identify. These include the family's beliefs about education and the ways that children learn, and hence the 'artificial environment' in the form of books or toys, computers or magnetic letters, they have created for their children's learning. They also include the family's relationship to their local community, to the wider society and to authority; their view of the world as a friendly and positive, or a threatening and negative, place to live in; and their confidence in their own abilities to manage their lives and make appropriate arrangements for their children. These underlying attitudes are communicated to young children in all kinds of ways, and help to shape the children's own attitudes. Both Sonia's and Saskia's home experiences are examples of this process, and of the consequences for children of different home cultures when they make their transitions out of the home.

Home culture and the 'habitus'

Some aspects of the environment that parents construct for their children are put in place very consciously: parents report that they have bought educational toys because they know that children learn through play, or have joined the library 'because it helps them with their reading' (Brooker 2002). Others are part of that unconscious provision which develops without any deliberate planning, because it is part of the parents' own early experiences: copying sentences out of books, reciting prayers or Bible texts, or naming the counting numbers. These practices all contribute to the unique but ephemeral culture of the home, which transforms a little with the arrival of each new family member, but retains many of its underlying beliefs and values.

It is this accumulation of beliefs, practices and attitudes which is described by Bourdieu (1990a) as the *habitus*, a set of dispositions towards life which informs what people say and do (and how they bring up their children). The *habitus* is shaped by any family's history, and geography, their social class and ethnicity, their experiences of education and employment, work and travel, and their social networks. Any or all of these factors may help to give families a positive or negative view of the world, including broadly optimistic or pessimistic expectations for their children, and a sense of their own efficacy as parents in achieving what they want for their children.

As children grow up in families, and hear adults talking and planning for their lives, they acquire some of these expectations and aspirations, and some of these beliefs about the nature of the world: as a trustworthy or untrustworthy, exciting or risky, place to be. According to Bourdieu, each child develops his or her own unique *habitus* because each child's experience is different, even within a single family: 'I am talking about dispositions *acquired through experience*, thus variable from place to place and time to time' (1990b: 9). But despite the uniqueness of each child's individual *habitus*, which changes over time as they encounter new experiences, some of the family's underlying attitudes inevitably contribute to it, and may persist throughout the child's life.

When we compare the early experiences of children like Saskia and Sonia, the concept of *habitus* helps to explain the 'cultural' differences in the psychosocial environments of their homes, and the expectations about the world that each of the little girls acquires there. Saskia, in her father's memorable phrase, has been taught that 'there's no shortage' of love and affection, care and companionship, pleasure and fun; that every transition she will make has a purpose and a logic in an essentially benevolent world; that all the new people she will meet will offer her the same security that she has experienced since birth. The family's positive attitudes to her nursery care givers prompts them to adopt nursery rituals at home, so that the whole family shares in and celebrates the little girl's experiences in her new environment. They make the transition together, not just by accompanying Saskia to nursery, but by including her world in the family culture, a culture shaped from positive and pleasurable experiences of life, work and social interactions. In doing so, they extend the family *habitus* to encompass new possibilities

The future appears rather different for Sonia and her family. 'Life' has not always treated them kindly, and Kath's childrearing efforts seem calculated to protect her children, as far as possible, from an untrustworthy and unreliable world. She has maintained a rather inward-looking household, avoiding contact with neighbours, and has kept the children at home in their pre-school years. Her own lack of success at school may have prompted her to instruct the children in the basics (colours, letters, numbers) when they were very young, and to require their siblings to do the same, to give them a better chance than she had. But her demeanour does not suggest much trust in the school as an institution, or in the teachers who welcome her into the classroom.

Given her own poor experience, Kath's belief that her children are not learning as much as she did is rather a sad one, but it is not something she will discuss with teachers. The barriers she has erected to protect her family from the outside world have also prevented her from forming the kind of links with the school which might boost Sonia's own trust and confidence. In marked contrast to Saskia's parents, she keeps her distance and keeps the dialogue to a minimum. As a result, there seems to be no place in Sonia's home for the culture of the classroom where she spends her days, while her home culture is not reflected in the school. The family *habitus*, which has developed from the experiences they have been through, does not encourage Sonia to welcome new experiences, trust new acquaintances, and take risks with new opportunities. Unlike

Saskia's, her transition to school is a relatively solitary adventure, fraught with anxieties.

The tools of the culture

If one significant aspect of the family (and child) *habitus* is an attitude to the world, and one's place in it, another is the kind of educational practice that takes place in the home. Returning to that early notion of culture as 'cultivation', or an environment for promoting growth and development, we must remember that an important aspect of the analogy is the need for appropriate tools. Whether for plants or humans, these tools have been, in Cole's (1998: 15) words 'perfected over generations and designed for the special tasks to which they were put'.

The tools of children's earliest education are many and varied. We are accustomed, thanks to Vygotsky (1962) to acknowledge that language itself is the pre-eminent cultural tool, and the means by which knowledge is constructed, assimilated and communicated. We know too, from decades of research, that the kinds of language children hear and acquire in their homes are not all equally valued in their classrooms (Bernstein 1971; Heath 1983; Michaels 1986). Not only bilingual children, but many monolingual English-speaking children, acquire their earliest knowledge and skills by means of a language which is significantly different from the language of teachers, and which does not serve them well when they make the transition to school (Tizard and Hughes 1984; Wells 1985).

But families provide other tools for children's learning, which are equally culturally specific. These may include spoons and forks, or chopsticks, as tools for eating; pens and pencils, or chubby crayons and finger paints, for mark-making; sacred texts, or cartoon books; construction toys or sewing kits; pop music videos or piano lessons; computer games or workbooks. Few families can afford all the educational tools they would like to provide for their children, but their choice of what to provide tells us a great deal about their understanding of development and learning. It also has a significant impact on the ease with which they make their transition into pre-school or school. As Barrett demonstrated in the 1980s, 'the match/mismatch of pupils' previous experience and knowledge, and that needed to engage with the experiences and expectations of school has been shown to be significant to how children respond in school' (1986: 115) This match and mismatch was described by Bourdieu in the 1970s, but is equally evident when some of today's children start school.

Learning at home

As the EPPE study has reminded us, it is not what parents *are*, but what they *do* with their children, which makes the difference in children's early acquisition of the cognitive and social skills which will help them to adapt to school (Sylva et al. 2004). This finding comes as an important warning against stereotyping: against the assumption that middle-class children will have had a more 'educative' home life than working-class children; or that ethnic minority parents have been less involved in their children's learning than white parents.

But there are of course connections between what parents 'are' and what they 'do', because their actions on the whole reflect both their goals for children, and their beliefs about the most effective ways to achieve these goals. These goals too may be entwined with beliefs and attitudes we could describe as 'cultural'. Parents who believe that learning is only achieved through hard work and memorization will not invest their time or money in educational toys and games. Parents who are less concerned with their daughters' learning than their sons' may make less investment in their girls. Parents who have never enjoyed reading themselves may struggle to find the time for reading with their children, though they may do all kinds of other things with them. The activities children undertake with their parents, from going fishing to hanging out the washing, will almost without exception be 'educational' as well as enjoyable, teaching knowledge and skills which most classrooms could never offer. But once they are enrolled in the education system, children's learning will follow another set of cultural guidelines, and the connections between home and school ideas of learning may become increasingly weak with each new transition children make.

Values and goals

Most childrearing practices are undertaken with specific, if unconscious, goals in mind. Parents from different cultural groups often hold different views of what an 'ideal child' looks like: an assertive, articulate, confident and independent individual, as in classic American studies, or a more submissive, supportive, interdependent member of a household, as in many studies of African and Asian families (Super and Harkness 1977). While western families typically encourage their children to engage in some kind of verbal dialogue from the moment they open their eyes, and view speaking as a major milestone in children's development, the children of families in the developing world may be encouraged instead to listen carefully, follow instructions, and take on responsibilities. Among the toddlers raised by the Kipsigis of Kenya, as Super and Harkness (1998) report, 'the rate of vocalisation ... is only half the American rate' and mothers 'do not see themselves as having a major role in "teaching" a child to talk': 'It is as though the parents' traditional attitude is that children will learn to talk soon enough on their own, but they must be taught to understand requests and instructions and to obey them. The parents' goal for young children is verbal comprehension, not production' (1998: 43–4).

Our own schools and pre-schools contain many children brought up by parents with similar goals. In the All Saints study (Brooker 2002), parents with an English background and upbringing all prioritized their children's ability to talk, chat, communicate, and generally express themselves; they rated 'being able to communicate' as the most important attribute for children starting school, and one which parents should try to foster. In the same neighbourhood, parents from Bangladeshi backgrounds rated this attribute very low in importance (on a scale of 1 to 5, most gave it 1), but they strongly emphasized their children's listening skills, and viewed this as a goal to work towards.

In our multicultural and globalized world, it is easy to see these two attributes – speaking and listening – not only as complementary, but as equally valid priorities for parenting. Yet our education system, on the whole, offers opportunities to children who can communicate, and assumes that those who are less talkative, less articulate, are at a disadvantage. This deficit view, however sympathetically held, may help to construct self-fulfilling prophecies.

Beliefs about learning

In addition to their diverse goals for children, parents may have differing opinions on how to achieve these goals. Most early years' practitioners will have found themselves complaining, at some time, about the pressure they receive from parents who want their children to 'work' rather than 'play' in their nursery and reception classes. Such pressures are reported from all kinds of parents, and for all kinds of reasons. There are middle-class parents who believe their child should be 'pushed' or 'stretched' (without stopping to consider the image these verbs actually conjure up); working-class parents who wish their children to be more successful academically than they themselves were, and who feel that starting formal work early is the best way to ensure this; ethnic minority families whose own school memories are of rote-learning and recitation, and who send their children to UK schools in the belief that the education will be 'better' than at home. Early years' practitioners frequently have to defend their own belief in the appropriateness of active, playful learning against parents' beliefs that formal learning offers their child a better chance of success.

However learning is provided for in the nursery or reception class, a child's understanding of 'how you learn' will have been acquired some time before, through their home experiences of all kinds of learning. In most homes, much of what children learn as babies and toddlers is implicit rather than explicit. Babies are rarely *told* how to talk or how to walk, and their cultural knowledge about the ways people behave with each other, and relate to each other, eat together and sleep together, are also learned through participation rather than through instruction. But as their understanding of language increases, their care givers' use of instructions grows with it: self-care skills such as feeding and dressing are learned through a complex process of demonstration, participation, trial and error and explanation.

Cross-cultural scholars have given detailed accounts of the way that young children are 'apprenticed' to the everyday behaviours of their culture and community (Rogoff 1990; Lave and Wenger 1991; Rogoff et al. 1993) including quite complex skills such as sewing and calligraphy. These accounts closely resemble the ways that the scaffolding of 'school' learning has been described: a process in which the task is broken down into small and manageable units; the adult helps the learner to focus on the tools and components needed for the next unit of the task; the adult offers physical or verbal support for the child, and then withdraws that support to allow the child to take control (Wood 1998).

Many parents, however, believe that the knowledge and skills needed for 'school' are learned by a different process: by adults presenting facts or techniques, which children then repeat, recite or imitate until they can reliably present the same set of facts or techniques back to the adult. These parents have good reason for their beliefs, which have under-pinned educational provision for centuries, and have penetrated to most parts of the world including those ex-colonial countries whose education system was laid down by European colonizers. In education as in other fields, like medicine, 'new knowledge' of the kind that has transformed European thought during the 20th century (from Piaget and Vygotsky, for instance) is slow to trickle down into the everyday or 'common-sense' knowledge which informs the family and community *habitus* of parents – what Bruner (1996) calls 'folk pedagogy'.

Research demonstrates again and again that this is so: we have the evidence of Bernstein's (1971) work with English mothers in the 1950s and 60s; of the Newsons' report on English working-class practices in the 1960s (Newson and Newson 1968, 1976); of Heath's work with

Appalachian families in the 70s and 80s; and of numerous studies of minority ethnic parents in the 80s and 90s (Ghuman and Gallop 1981; Ghuman and Wong 1989; Gregory and Biarnes 1994). The All Saints study (Brooker 2002) confirmed what practitioners know: that faith in traditional methods of rote learning is still strong among many groups. As parents explain, this is how they learned, and it worked for them, so why should their children not benefit from the same methods?

Preparing them for school

The occasion of a child starting in nursery or reception is an anxious time for families because they have anticipated it ever since the child was small. For parents, their children's early years always have this milestone ahead, to look forward to but also to fear a little, and studies show that it is common for a great deal of thought to go into preparing the child for school over the weeks, months and even years before they start.

Cleave et al. (1982), in one of the earliest studies of transition, reported a range of attitudes and behaviours among parents. One group of parents 'viewed the transfer with some trepidation and were deliberately playing it down so as not to put the child off' (1982: 95), while others used the 'hard work' and 'reading and writing' children would encounter in the classroom as either a threat or a promise. On the whole, parents in this study agreed that the purposes of school were completely different from those of pre-school. They explained to the researchers that 'Of course one is a play school and the other is a learning school'; that pre-school staff simply 'supervise their play' and 'keep them amused' while school staff 'get cracking with teaching them' and 'have to keep up standards' (1982: 92). Recent studies show that similar concerns are still felt (and are communicated to children).

In the All Saints' study (Brooker 2002) parents' beliefs and behaviours were accounted for by each family's particular *habitus*. The parents brought up in rural Bangladesh, without exception, told their children that they would need to 'study' from the first day in reception. In preparing them for school, they instructed their children to 'sit still', 'say nothing', 'listen to the teacher and study hard'. They explained that the English education system was the principal reason they had left their homeland, and they wanted their children to excel within it. They believed that their children started school with a disadvantage, not only because of their limited English, but because they as parents could not give them all the support they would like to. In consequence they emphasized that their children must not waste time in play, but must work hard every day.

Among parents in the same neighbourhood with an English education, feelings were mixed. Most families had heard it said that children 'learned through play', but they were not completely convinced of this, and were heartily relieved if they saw some signs that their children were 'working'. Even those with experience of running playgroups or attending family drop-ins, who were most tolerant of play as a strategy for children's learning, did not seem convinced of its effectiveness. One of these mothers explained in an interview that 'children should be allowed to play a lot at first, and then learn more, bit by bit' (Brooker 2002: 53). Parents with older children in the school were more relaxed about the pace of learning, although the minority of mothers who had done badly at school themselves were more inclined to be anxious about their child's success, and less inclined to leave it to chance.

Families, like Saskia's, who are confident about their own lives, and their child's future can afford to feel relaxed about the child's early experiences, and to prioritize fun and happiness. It is hard to imagine Saskia's parents encouraging her to read dictionaries before starting school. But families who lack confidence in their child's ability to succeed may legitimately wish to force the pace, to give their child a head start in an environment where they feel the odds are stacked against them. Part of the *habitus*, as Bourdieu describes it, is defined by the kinds of strategies parents deploy in working towards their children's future success. Preparing children for school involves some key decisions about acting strategically, because parents as well as teachers know that this transition will have lasting consequences. And much of this strategic thinking revolves around their understanding of readiness.

'Ready to learn' in school and pre-school

Small-scale studies of the ways that families bring up their children and prepare them for school can be contextualized by the large-scale surveys of school readiness beliefs which have been reported from all parts of the world. Despite many individual, local and regional variations, some broad trends emerge very clearly about the relationship between 'home' and 'school' aims for children at the time of transition.

Global trends

There appears to be a consensus, in transition studies from around the world, that parents, pre-school teachers and school teachers of children aged 3 to 7 hold somewhat different views of what constitutes 'readiness' as children start their education. A wide-ranging review of these studies, conducted for UNESCO (Arnold et al. 2006), summarizes a situation that is found just as commonly in rural communities in Asia and Africa as it is in the affluent western nations: 'educators and parents often have different definitions of school readiness. Teachers put more emphasis on the social domain whereas many parents emphasize academic readiness' (Arnold et al. 2006: 7). But the report goes on to cite evidence that, where children have participated in early childhood programmes, parents' priorities are seen to change:

> Examples abound from programmes serving low-income rural families ... in which parents who had clearly demanded 'school learning' in the beginning are in reality most appreciative of their children's social development. They delight in their children's cleverness but talk most about the fact that they are polite, respectful, obedient and friendly and, at the same time, confident, curious and comfortable even with new people. They appear to combine traits that have traditionally been emphasized for children within the culture with those that are critical for coping with a changing world.
>
> (Arnold et al. 2006: 7)

In other words, parents' cultural beliefs and theories about learning sometimes change in response to their children's early experiences.

At a global level, the report finds, the consensus from educators is that children's readiness has five domains: physical well-being and motor development; social and emotional development; language development; cognition and general knowledge; and 'approaches to learning', or positive dispositions. Though few educators, or parents, would argue with this list, it is evident that the domains are interpreted differently by the different groups involved with children. In many developing regions, physical well-being, in terms of nutrition, hygiene and favourable conditions for growth and survival, take priority over all the other domains, whereas this pre-condition is achieved without special interventions in most parts of the western world. Once physical development is assured, the attentions of care givers seem to focus on either the social or the cognitive domains, with most parents highlighting academic or cognitive skills.

Readiness and resources: the USA

In the United States, readiness was a key concept in the large-scale programmes set up to improve the school performance of children who had been enrolled in programmes like Head Start (Kagan and Neuman 1998; Ramey et al. 1998). Concern over the 'wash-out' of children's early gains in cognitive development resulted in a series of transition programmes, and a set of National Goals for Education, the first of which stated that: 'All children in America will start school ready to learn' (National Education Goals Panel 1991).

A study by Piotrkowski et al. (2000), which surveyed the views on school readiness of different stakeholder groups in a large and very poor American school district, confirmed the 'global' trends in perspectives, but also explored the underlying rationale for them. In this district, both parents and educators agreed on the need for children to be healthy and socially competent, but the parents, who believed that a child's 'knowledge' was more important than their approach to learning, valued academic skills much more highly than their children's educators. The researchers explain the rationale for the parents' views by importantly redefining 'school readiness' as a concept which is wider than the individual child. Readiness is defined instead as 'the social, political, organizational, educational and personal *resources* that support children's success at school entry' (2000: 540). These resources are identified at four different levels: at the 'neighbourhood level', which includes resources such as high-quality day care and pre-school provision, libraries and playgrounds; at the 'local' level, which includes resources such as parent involvement programmes, professional development for teachers and strong educational leadership; at the 'family level', which includes parents' childrearing skills as well as their own education and levels of poverty; and at the individual 'child level' which includes the domains of physical and social development that are described in global reports.

What this means is that the *resourcefulness* of individual children is situated in the resourcefulness of their environment. As Piotrkowski emphasizes, in communities where the neighbourhood and local resources are poor, such as inner-city ghettoes, a child's future chances depend far more on the resources possessed by the family and child. Parents know this, he suggests (if only intuitively), and in consequence place far more emphasis on the child's early academic learning in the home. If they know too that their family resources are poor, such that the 'home learning environment' described by the EPPE study (Sylva et al. 2004) is of poor quality, they will exercise even more pressure to ensure that their child is introduced to formal learning, and encouraged to 'work hard', in the pre-school setting and at the start of school. In other words,

local school and family readiness resources influence beliefs about what children should know and be able to do at kindergarten entry.

> In economically depressed communities ... parents' elevated
> readiness beliefs regarding the resources children need for
> kindergarten may be a function not of developmentally
> inappropriate expectations but of realistic concerns that their
> children might not succeed in resource-poor local schools.
>
> (Piotrkowski et al. 2000: 554)

These very plausible conclusions help to explain the beliefs reported in
many studies of low-income or ethnic-minority families, who know their
children are 'resource poor' at some levels, and wish to compensate by
promoting the academic resources of the individual child.

Parents' views are supported by evidence from educators. In their
survey of 10,000 kindergarten teachers, Rimm-Kaufman et al. (2000)
reported that the most common problems named by teachers were
'difficulty following directions' and 'lack of academic skills'; and that
these problems were described as more serious if the school drew pupils
from poor and ethnic-minority communities. For all the educators'
explicit emphasis on social development, it seems as if poor parents are
correct in identifying academic skills as the key to their children's
smooth transition to school, and future progress. Sonia's family could
certainly be included in this category.

Australian views of readiness

Comparable evidence on the 'readiness' beliefs of parents and educators
in Australia, are provided by a long-term study of starting school
(Dockett and Perry, 2002, 2004, 2005). In designing one survey, the
authors pointed out that, in their experience of talking to parents, 'definitions of readiness vary, as do the ways of assessing readiness. Often,
comments are made about children's ages, gender, maturity and physical
stature' (Dockett and Perry 2002: 68). Their own questionnaire, rather
than offering parents and educators categories to choose from, gave the
very open invitation: 'List the first five things that come into your mind
when you think about a child starting school'. Both groups of adults cited
aspects of 'adjustment' or 'adaptation' far more frequently than any
specific aspects of knowledge or skills: they wanted children to fit in,
make friends and feel comfortable, and they understood that their academic progress would depend on this sense of well-being. One teacher is
quoted as saying, 'I can teach them to read and write, so they don't need
to know that before they start. I want kids who are happy and want to be
here' (Dockett and Perry 2002: 82).

At the moment of transition, 'happiness' is at the top of the agenda for both parents and educators. But when a subsequent survey asked these two groups to rate the signs of a successful transition, the characteristic divide between parents and teachers reappears: 'parents rated items reflecting knowledge as more important than teachers ... Teachers in schools rated items reflecting adjustment and disposition as more important than parents' (Dockett and Perry 2004: 227). As the authors point out, a lack of shared understandings of what matters most *during* children's transition period makes continuing communication and collaboration problematic as the child moves on through the education system.

Conclusion: *bridges and barriers*

This chapter has discussed the effects on children of moving from one culture, that of the home and community, to another, that of the world of early childhood education. We have seen that the barriers between home and school for many children are barriers of beliefs as well as practices: the contrast between the ideology of schools and settings, and the beliefs enshrined in the family *habitus*, can result in children seeming unsuitable and lacking in resources in the classroom. The task of educators, of course, is to build bridges over these barriers, by constructing relationships with the home care givers which provide a friendly and welcoming space for children to explore new experiences and new roles, with maximum support for their efforts.

At home, as in their pre-school and school settings, children inhabit 'cultures': environments designed by adults for their care and education in general, and with specific goals and objectives, conscious or unconscious, in mind. These environments may be equally appropriate for their growth and development, and the aim of successful transitions must be that the child will feel an equally strong sense of belonging and well-being in both. Moving into educational settings does not mean leaving your family or community behind – as Saskia's dad pointed out, 'there's no shortage ... we're still here!' – and children like Saskia reap the benefits of environments which are complementary. When a good match between two settings is established, the potential for development, as well as for the child's happiness, is enormous.

The characteristics of the home culture, and home *habitus*, as we have seen, reflect the social class and ethnic identity of the family, as well as its particular history of education and employment, and its ongoing relationship with the outside world, in the shape of the community, neighbourhood and wider society. These characteristics shape parents' values and goals for children, and their beliefs about the best way to achieve them. One aspect of these beliefs includes an idea about readiness: what do children need to know and do, in order to be 'ready to learn' or 'ready for school'? Another is parents' evaluation of the resources available to children as they get ready for school.

The whole question of the readiness of schools for children will be discussed in the next chapter, which looks at the continuities and discontinuities which children face as they make their transitions within the education system. But we should remember here that Bronfenbrenner's description of children's place in the ecosystem looks beyond their immediate experience of microsystems and mesosystems to consider the impact of national and other structures. Bronfenbrenner also described a *macrosystem* at the level of society as a whole – government policies and national ideologies – which children are unaware of, but which provides a blueprint for all the smaller systems they might encounter in their everyday lives (early years policies, childcare policies, family policies). And there are also *exosystems*: those mysterious locations which shape the lives of parents and other adults, invisible to children but with a potential impact on their lives (parents' places of employment or study; welfare agencies; health facilities; community associations). In considering children's transitions, we need to be aware, not just of their immediate circumstances, but of the more hidden policy decisions and institutions which combine to build the structures within which the child and family acquire their resources and their resilience. These too are part of the visible and invisible culture of the child.

4

Continuities: stepping up through the system

I felt scared because I did not know my teacher. I did not see any sand area, or a carpentry corner, not even a see-saw or a swing. The environment looked strange to me. My teacher gave orders to us and we had to move quickly or else. I thought of pre-school. I did not want to come back the next day. I asked my mother to take me back to pre-school. My mother told me my age is not to be at pre-school but at class one in the school.

(School pupil, Fiji)

I think that we must learn to use the transitions in children's lives far more positively, with greater insight into their potential, rather than seeing transitions as problematic for every child.

(Bennett 2006: 15)

As we have seen, homes, schools and other settings for young children can all be thought of as cultures, providing 'environments for the optimal growth and development of the young', and the first transition from home into the education system is often regarded as the biggest 'culture shock' a child will encounter. Traditionally, this particular move is seen as the one which most challenges children's courage and resilience. But on reflection we may feel this is mistaken; because whereas children's early transitions are generally planned and managed with tremendous care, subsequent transitions – *within* the system – are often less well supported.

This chapter is concerned with the transitions children undertake as they 'move up' through the education system. There are many such transitions, and they vary according to the policies of the country, state, district or even school that the child is entering – from under-3s to over-3s, from pre-school to Reception, from Foundation Stage Unit to Year 1; or from pre-K to Kindergarten and then to first grade in the USA and elsewhere. Within this complex picture of systems and settings, a single key moment stands out: almost every child, in almost every location, will encounter at some point the irreversible change from informal to formal learning that characterizes most education systems.

Informal learning – 'child friendly', 'child initiated', 'play based' and 'hands on' – is the key characteristic of early years' education, and is a principle that has been vigorously defended over the hundred years or more that nursery education has been provided. Despite occasional skirmishes, this battle has now been won, in many parts of the world. In England, the *Practice Guidance for the Early Years Foundation Stage* (DfES 2007: 7), which regulates all provision for children from birth to 5, states unequivocally that 'Play underpins all development and learning for young children ... and it is through play that they develop intellectually, creatively, physically, socially and emotionally'. The unspoken assumption is that children develop and learn in a completely different way after the age of 5, and this is when children may discover that their readiness for school is ill-matched with the school's readiness for them.

An international consensus on the importance of 'active, play-based pedagogy' was identified in Bertram and Pascal's (2002: ii) review of the early years' provision in 20 countries, ranging from Western Europe to Japan and Korea, New Zealand and Australia. Not surprisingly, almost all the participants in this seminar project were also concerned with improving the transition from early years' settings to primary school, a concern reflected in the statement that 'the separation between early years and primary education ... caused some level of discontinuity in most participating countries' (2002: 42).

This chapter addresses the issue of 'discontinuity', but emphasizes the solutions rather than the problems. It describes first the ways that two children with particular needs – one diagnosed with autistic spectrum disorder, and one identified as 'gifted and talented' – were supported in the transition from pre-school to school. A review of research on 'transitions within the system', and of the structural arrangements which contribute to discontinuities, is followed by a consideration of the risk factors and protective factors for children undergoing transitions. Above all it is clear that a good pre-school experience can endow children with the *resilience* they will require to cope with discontinuities, the *resources* they need for formal learning, and the *reciprocity* which will keep them actively engaged in a learning community. Finally, I offer examples of transitions projects which have successfully bridged the divides between phases.

Case studies in cross-phase transitions: Harry and Louis

Harry, from a rural area in England, and Louis, from Central London, were both identified by their pre-school care givers as having additional needs which would require careful support during their transition to primary school. Their stories show how practitioners, working with parents, can provide the resources children need to sustain them as they cross the bridge between phases.

Harry's story

Harry began attending a crèche at his mum's place of work when he was a baby, and continued there when he was subsequently enrolled in another nursery near to his home. Just before his third birthday he underwent a multi-disciplinary assessment and was identified as having a form of autism, and given a statement of Special Educational Needs which entitled him to additional individual support for a few hours a week during his two remaining years in his nursery settings. His mum reported that 'Harry is settled and very happy in both the nursery settings that he attends so, since his delayed development became apparent, my overriding concern has been the transition to school'. Fortunately for Harry, his local education authority was piloting a systematic transitions framework which seemed designed to meet his needs.

Plans for Harry's transition to primary school involved a number of people: the staff from both the nurseries he attended, including his own support worker, his parents, the area Special Needs Coordinator (SENCO), an area Autism Support Worker, a speech therapist and the staff of the school where he was due to start in the following September. The size of the team created some difficulties in organizing joint meetings, but these were overcome with careful planning. The first joint meeting took place at the new school in the spring before he was due to start, and the process of preparing Harry for change began soon afterwards. As one of his nursery teachers wrote in her report, 'We know Harry, Harry knows us, the school does not know Harry and Harry does not like change of routine, place or people'. It was clear that Harry would need additional resources in order to cope with the transition.

Harry's current support worker began to accompany him on a series of visits to his new school during the summer term, helping him to get used to the environment, and identifying the aspects of it which caused him anxiety. Together they got to know the new support worker who would assume responsibility for Harry's additional needs in his primary classroom. At around the same time, the Reception teacher visited the nursery to meet Harry in his familiar surroundings, and share the photographic records and observations that the staff there had compiled. Since the long summer holiday was to intervene before Harry actually started school, arrangements were also made for Harry's mum to have a set of photographs of the new setting, to discuss with him during the summer, and for them to pop in to the school grounds from time to time to enhance Harry's familiarity. The final arrangement was for a special book to be prepared for Harry by his prospective teachers, with photos of his tray, peg, work area, dining area and all the other new sights he would need to manage. By this time Harry's mum, and all the practitioners working with him, had established strong links which would enable Harry to experience the maximum continuity between settings as he began his formal school career.

Louis's story

Louis started nursery in a busy London nursery school, in a neighbourhood whose mixed population included the highly affluent and the extremely poor – both well-known media professionals and recently arrived asylum-seekers. The headteacher's concern, for many of her children, was that their range of socioeconomic and cultural backgrounds, and the varied level of their curriculum achievements, appeared to mask their extraordinarily varied talents and skills once they moved from nursery into primary school. While the nursery staff agreed that a high proportion of their children appeared to have 'special' skills and talents, the children's receiving teachers apparently had fewer opportunities to notice and build on these once they started primary school. The nursery therefore embarked on a 'Gifted & Talented' project, a piece of action research designed to identify children's strengths across a wide spectrum of qualities, and in collaboration with parents; and then to liaise with primary schools in ways which would help the children's new teachers to be more aware of these qualities, and if possible to build on them.

The school adapted an identification tool, the 'Starry Night Protocol' (Gagne 1991; Eyre 1997) and used it to screen all the children who would be leaving the school in one 12-month period. Louis was one of these. Their protocol featured 12 'constellations' of behaviour, including 'sees the big picture' (comprehends, associates, predicts, analyses, theorizes); 'sensitive' (expressive, insightful, helpful, sympathetic/empathetic); 'imagery' (uses metaphors, detects symbolism, illustrates, expresses); and 'humour' (enjoys jokes, reacts and responds, notices and creates). Louis's profile was completed by his key worker and his mother, and the headteacher subsequently held a meeting with his parents, in which to discuss his outstanding qualities, and hear how they felt about Louis's imminent transition to school.

Louis's profile showed some areas of agreement between his key worker and his mother: both gave him high ratings for humour, curiosity, vocabulary and recall, although his mother also felt he was outstanding in empathy and imagination, while his key worker was uncertain about these qualities. Both could also identify areas of potential vulnerability: Louis's strong personality, and his highly idiosyncratic ideas and initiatives were easily catered for in the nursery but might be less well appreciated in a Reception class. As the transition approached, and with everyone's agreement, the portfolio containing Louis's profile was passed to the reception teacher, who agreed to monitor and report on his progress to both parents and nursery.

In the follow-up, the Reception teacher – like others involved in the project – expressed very positive feelings about the liaison process, and the information in the profile. Louis, she said 'was correctly identified by yourselves, and definitely sticks out amongst his peers ... This child's curiosity and outlandish questions are a real challenge to satisfy – we try and see it as a strength but it is hard with the formal demands of the curriculum'. Louis's transition from an environment where he could simply be himself, to one in which greater conformity was required, was never going to be straightforward but the positive and constructive view of him which this liaison created helped to set him on a trajectory in which his strengths were recognized, and allowances were made.

Stepping-up through the early years

Both Harry and Louis had the support of pre-school and school practitioners who ensured that their individuality was appreciated, and that they themselves would be as 'suitable' in their school class as they had been in their nurseries. Not all children are as fortunate. Educators as well as parents acknowledge that children benefit from more formal learning environments, and more abstract learning experiences, as they develop, and no one would suggest that children should remain indefinitely in nursery-style environments. But it is the suddenness of the shift, and the age at which it occurs, that has preoccupied researchers over the last decade. The 'discontinuities' that are frequently experienced are felt by parents as well as children, and increasing efforts have been made to address them at the level of policy and practice (Kagan and Neuman 1998; Fabian and Dunlop 2006).

Two steps to formal learning?

One consequence of these concerns about the shift to formal learning has been the increased provision of intermediate and preparatory classes. England has always had its 'reception classes', which children entered before reaching statutory school age, and the USA its kindergarten year, which is still not mandatory everywhere. But in recent years many European countries, with later starting ages for statutory schooling, have introduced a pre-primary year intended to accustom children to some of the requirements of school: a preparatory year in which school subjects and school routines are introduced but without the formality of the later school years (Bertram and Pascal 2002; Bennett 2006).

This half-way house to formal learning, which is intended to make transition more gradual, raises its own questions as we have seen in the debates over the appropriate provision for Reception children in England (Quick et al. 2002). Early years practitioners argue with passion that Reception children, aged 4 to 5, should be exempt from formal instruction and assessment until they have moved into Year 1 and beyond. They report, however, that the downward pressure of the National Curriculum, or pressure from parents, obliges them to make increasingly formal provision, especially for literacy and numeracy, long before this. With individual education authorities, and schools, making their own interpretations of the curriculum requirements, some English children may begin a desk-based learning experience from their fourth birthday, while others may experience a play-based pedagogy until well after they are 5. In consequence parents, as well as children, may feel they are 'starting school' twice over – once on entry to Reception and a second time, a year later, on entry to Year 1.

Stepping up through kindergarten: learning from the US experience

Similar repeat-moves are the focus of the major American studies, which began by exploring the transition to kindergarten (from pre-school or more specifically from Head Start), and have focused more recently on the transition from kindergarten into First Grade.

Kagan and Neuman (1998) reviewed the 'lessons' learned from three decades of research into the former of these, and argued that there was little evidence of progress during that period. Despite some examples of good practice, they found that only a minority of settings built on children's previous experiences and knowledge, and few valued the culture and learning children had acquired in their homes. Interventions such as the Head Start Transition project (1985) showed beneficial outcomes – more resilience among children, and more positive responses from teachers – but these successes were rarely replicated, and national studies showed that few of the school districts surveyed made any provision for transition. A subsequent national survey of kindergarten teachers' views concluded that there was 'a poor "fit" between children's competencies and aspects of the kindergarten classroom context, including teachers' expectations and classroom demands' (Rimm-Kaufman et al. 2000: 163).

Studies of the transition from Kindergarten to First Grade showed similar results: on the one hand, a poor profile of good practice at the national level, but on the other some positive outcomes from schools and districts which had made efforts at intervention (Entwisle and Alexander 1998; La Paro et al. 2000). By the time children reached the age of 6, very few schools were involving parents in their child's transition, and the majority simply passed on record cards and curriculum information. As La Paro (2000: 75) reported, typical American practices 'represent a fairly low-intensity and non-individualized approach to the transitions and do not involve the family'.

An evaluation by Mangione and Speth (1998) gave a more encouraging example. They described a 'framework for continuity' developed within one Californian community, to link schools, pre-schools, community settings and all the other services used by families with young children. One feature of the framework is a 'stepping-up ceremony', attended by almost all families and practitioners as well as local officials, to mark children's transition from their pre-schools (run by black community groups) to their schools (run by the white school district). The ceremony itself symbolized a shift in attitude on the part of all those involved, and affirmed the importance of their partnership within the framework:

> As important as the joint participation of the preschool and the elementary school in the preschool graduation was, everyone present considered the day-to-day work of the partnership more important. They shared the belief that a smooth transition to school depended on the support the community's children and families received before and after school entry.
>
> (1998: 392)

The final evaluation of this innovative project showed a consensus among participants that 'starting school' must be viewed as part of a long-term relationship between all those involved in the child's well-being:

> Respondents working in elementary schools feel just as strongly as professionals in early childhood education, social services and health-related fields that the framework appropriately places the transition to school within the broad context of early childhood continuity and home, school and community partnerships.
>
> (1998: 394)

What do they expect? Parents, pre-school teachers and teachers

The importance of a well-established partnership, such as that described by Mangione and Speth (1998), is very evident when we see the extent of the misunderstandings between parents, pre-school teachers and 'school' teachers which other studies portray. The researcher Stig Broström (2002) undertook a comparison between Danish pre-school and school teachers, and those reported in the main American studies, and concluded that similar barriers to understanding were present in the two societies. Danish pre-school teachers, he argues, believe (wrongly) that children will sit at desks all day once they start school, while school teachers have only the vaguest idea of the purposes and practice of pre-schools. The two groups have different ideas about what makes children 'ready for school', but rarely communicate with each other in ways which might bridge their perspectives. In consequence many children are mis-informed before their transition, and express unrealistic and outdated expectations, or at best are vague about what lies ahead. In consequence, Broström reports, many are anxious and fearful.

In an effort to reduce these misunderstandings, Broström (2002) went on to investigate the kinds of resources which were being offered to children within the Danish system, and to evaluate their effectiveness. His survey, designed to see which of 32 transition practices were most popular, was sent to pre-school teachers (called rather confusingly Kindergarten teachers), reception teachers (called Kindergarten Class teachers), and teachers from the first and second grades of school and the after-school provision. By far the most popular activities were those in which the pre-school child, or the whole class, visited the school classroom, or the school teacher paid a visit to the pre-school. Very few activities were undertaken which addressed the child as an individual rather than as a member of a cohort, or which involved parents in a visit or home visit. And whereas the participants in the American comparison studies were on the whole keen to develop more curriculum continuity, this idea was not popular with the Danish teachers, who saw the school and pre-school spheres as quite separate.

Similar differences are found everywhere, as Arnold and et al. (2006) identified. For all their local and cultural differences, education systems globally have evolved a view of the child as an entity who changes rather suddenly, at the age of 4 or 5 or 6, from someone who learns best through play and self-initiated activities into someone suited to formal instruction; from someone whose overall development, including their social and emotional aspects, requires holistic care, to someone whose cognitive development can be addressed in relative isolation. The study of English adults' views of children, referred to earlier (Hendy and Whitebread 2000) shows this with great clarity, but reveals too that children's competence, and their ability to construct their own learning, is increasingly under-estimated as the child moves through the school years. Our competent nursery children may turn into incompetent learners as they adapt to the school environment, and the experience of school 'dissuades them from independent action, towards a dependency relationship with their teachers' (Hendy and Whitebread 2000: 251).

Fortunately for such children, the evidence is increasing that a high-quality early years experience – one which strengthens the 3 Rs – acts as a protective factor during the discontinuities that follow. The 'risks' resulting from these discontinuities are highlighted by studies of children's anxieties over many different aspects of school cultures: structural and curricular, social and emotional.

Risk factors from discontinuities

Understanding time and space

As most studies show, moving into formal schooling generally involves moving to a larger and more complex building, in which it is easy to lose one's way. At the same time children are often moving from an integrated experience, in which all activities and facilities – meals and snacks, toilets and washrooms, music and dance, art and ICT – are located in a small area and within sight, to a more segregated experience in which they are required to present themselves in different parts of the building for different activities. 'Playtime', lunch time, PE, assembly, singing and other features of the timetable may be located some way from the classroom, while accessing the toilets and washrooms may be a particularly tough challenge for children who are already anxious, confused or fearful of doing something wrong.

Changes of place and space may be compounded by temporal changes. Paradoxically, traditional concerns about the 'long school day' experienced by children on starting school are now matched by concerns about the *shorter* day in school which contrasts with the extended-day nursery many children have known. Children may graduate from a long-day nursery place into half-day schooling during their first term, and have to handle additional moves into before-school and after-school care at the same time. On top of this the time spent *in school* may be divided into so many separate lessons and tasks that many different horizontal transitions are required. Skinner et al. (1998), who studied children's experience of transition in 14 different US classrooms, describe a marked emphasis by teachers on the demarcation of time and space, and of appropriate activities and behaviours. Typically, they found

> teachers carved up the school day into discrete times: arrival time, calendar time, math time, reading time, circle time, snack time, playground time, lunch time, story time, bathroom time, sharing time, nap time, review time and so forth ... In terms of both space and time, children were required to make a number of transitions throughout the day.
>
> (1998: 301)

Skinner argues that such 'over-differentiation' of time and place during the school day creates additional difficulties for children with special needs, or from minority ethnic backgrounds, who may have had no prior warning of how the school day was constructed, or who may lack a good grasp of routines.

Organizational matters: the 'rules' of school

While discontinuities in curriculum are often criticized by adults, it must be remembered that, from a child's perspective, the introduction of a new subject-based curriculum may be one of the anticipated treats of 'big school', and many children are proud to announce that they have to 'do literacy' and 'hard work' in their new class (O'Kane and Hayes 2007). Although pre-school practitioners continue to advocate an integrated approach to learning, the novelty of studying history, geography, science and even 'phonics' can hold great charms for children, at least initially.

A more serious impact on children's attitude to their learning – the all-important dispositions to enquire, explore and persist with difficulties – derives from a change in pedagogy, and in children's loss of control over their learning environment. As Cleave et al. (1982) pointed out, the move to formal schooling is typically a move from child-initiated and child-directed activities, where up to 70 per cent of the day may be controlled by the child, to adult-initiated and adult-directed activities, where as little as 20 per cent of the time is controlled by the child. These percentages, they added, disguise the fact that the adult-controlled parts of the pre school day may have been 'fun' times such as stories and action songs. Barrett (1989) argued that children's discovery of the implications of 'work' and 'play' in primary school could lead to disaffection from an early age.

In Skinner's study, the frequent horizontal transitions of the kindergarten classroom were accomplished by means of management strategies which the children found equally confusing, as they were asked to 'freeze' on a given signal, and then abandon the activity they were involved in and move to a new one. Teachers worked hard to inculcate the appropriate behaviours for these transitions, using circle times to discuss rules for sitting, standing, sharing, turn taking and so on. As the authors comment,

> Over the years, teachers had constructed rules for nearly every space and activity in the classroom and wider school environs: rules that made shifting between activities go more smoothly, and behaviour management strategies that helped the children stay focused and out of trouble and kept the teachers from losing power and control.
>
> (Skinner et al. 1998: 302)

In these classrooms, children who 'behaved' were commended, while those who achieved academically but did not comply were characterized as 'immature', 'unfocused' and as 'having an attitude'; failure in this latter sphere was attributed to 'lack of structure in the home' (Skinner et al. 1998: 304) but may have been due to difficulties in adjusting to unfamiliar expectations. A similar case is made by Entwisle and Alexander:

> Children who slip easily into the student role enhance their own development. A child who has the temperament and inclination to fit in well gets better marks and gains more on standardized tests in the early grades than does a child who has fewer of those qualities.
>
> (1998: 353)

Evidence of this kind confirms the importance of transitional support for children like Harry and Louis, who may not have made a good impression on their teachers without it.

Changes in identity

The transition from a small pre-school to a larger school brings with it a dramatic enlargement of the child's social experience: not just strange adults, but large numbers of adults, whose names are easily mis-remembered or mixed up; not just new children, but huge hordes of new children who are also *big* children.

The shift in identity which occurs when a child moves from being among the oldest and biggest people in a small setting, to being one of the youngest and smallest people in a large setting, can be dramatic. The discovery of the highly relative quality of terms like 'big' and 'small' may be conceptually challenging too: many mothers interviewed for the All Saints' study (Brooker 2002) explained that they had told their children they would be going to school 'because they were big now', whereas the children's first actual experience of school showed them that the reverse was true. (Teachers as well as parents may contribute to this sense of dislocation: in the Valley School study (Brooker 1996), the 4-year-old nursery 'graduates' who had so impressed me with their maturity during research interviews were referred to in their first school assembly as 'the babies' by a headteacher who was trying to impress on the older children the importance of looking after them.) Children's own accounts of this change in status are discussed in Chapter 5.

Every transition into a new group challenges our sense of identity, and successive experiences teach us strategies for coping with the challenge. Research indicates that children who mixed freely with peers of the opposite sex, or of other ethnic groups, in their previous or pre-school environment, often seek security by adherence to a gendered or racia-lized group identity as a result of transition (Jackson and Warin 2000; Corsaro 2003; Brooker 2006). This natural tendency to seek safety inside an in-group may have unwanted consequences, as children relinquish valuable friendships, and pursue increasingly stereotyped behaviours and attitudes.

Discontinuities: protective factors

Fortunately, the 'risk factors' in the shift into formal learning environments are matched by a range of protective factors, which enable most children to respond well to new challenges. The value of high-quality early experiences, as we now know without doubt, is revealed in the way that children demonstrate the necessary resilience to settle and succeed in their new environments. If certain important characteristics are put in place in the pre-school environment, they persist as long-term dispositions.

Promoting resilience

> The identification of protective factors has led to preventive approaches to equip children with competencies to meet future demands ... children can not turn into resilient persons by themselves. They need significant support from their social systems.
>
> (Niesel and Griebel 2005: 4, 6)

Resilience, generally understood as the ability to develop normally in adverse circumstances (Fonagy et al. 1994), is no longer regarded as an innate and stable characteristic of children, but as a quality which can be strengthened and supported by adult intervention. Resilient children are those who are generally optimistic about their abilities and about the likelihood of succeeding; who actively seek solutions to problems, including resolving conflicts and disagreements; and who have an internal 'locus of control' which enables them to be self-reliant rather than depending on others. One of their strengths is their ability to engage with others and mobilize social networks – their *reciprocity* – and so to make creative use of all the human as well as material resources to hand – their *resourcefulness*. In everyday life in the classroom, we may identify them as the kinds of children who announce that they 'have a good idea' for an activity or for solving a problem, and co-opt other children and adults, and all the available resources, to put their idea into action.

In common with other desirable dispositions, resilience can not be 'taught' but it can be facilitated and strengthened by positive pre-school experiences.

- Educators *can* teach children to identify problems and think logically and creatively about their solution. Such 'problems' are frequently not merely physical, but social and emotional: sharing and turn taking, developing empathy, adopting a variety of perspectives and considering a range of options and outcomes.
- Children *can* be taught the benefits of working collaboratively, listening to each other, and taking responsibility for their group and their environment. Participating in shared activities, and communicating with others about their plans and projects, enhances children's self-esteem and initiates a virtuous circle in which the individual child's resilience is both confirmed, and communicated to other children. (Rutter 2000; Niesel and Griebel 2005).

Relationships and friendships

Making relationships, with peers and adults, is a key task for children in the pre-school years, and friends are an important resource during transitions. As Trevarthen (1998: 97) points out, 'A three-year-old is a socially aware person who is capable of making and keeping friends and of negotiating interesting co-operations and tests of understandings with a wide range of acquaintances'.

By the time they leave pre-school most children have experienced a range of peer relationships, and many have constructed friendships which persist through the transition into school, providing them with 'the emotional and cognitive resources necessary for successful adaptation to their [new] social world' (Faulkner and Miell 1993: 25). Small-scale studies show that stepping up through the school system is often easier for children with existing friends: 'Compared to children without friends, children with friends in the classroom during the first weeks developed more positive views of school' (Broström 2002: 56). The All Saints' study (Brooker 2002) found that children who had a friend from pre-school, or a neighbour's child, in their reception class soon showed high levels of involvement in learning activities, in comparison with those who started school without a friend: the latter group were more likely to hover, wait and watch during their early weeks in the classroom.

Corsaro in a lengthy study of Italian children's transitions to school, argued that adults must 'understand the dynamic quality of children's friendships, especially as these change after a transition to a new school' (2003: 290). His observations showed that having a friend enabled a child to 'remain themselves' – to hang on to their existing identity – rather than having to carve out a new identity, which was more likely to be constrained by classroom stereotypes about gender, age and ethnicity.

Children who 'lose' friends when they change classrooms are likely to feel helpless and vulnerable, so it is important for teachers to work with both pre-school teachers and parents to ensure that this is avoided as far as possible. Children's own views on this subject are further explored in Chapter 5.

Family factors

The strongest resource available to most children during transitions will be their own family experience and the preparatory work of parents, who can support children in becoming resilient and resourceful, and in forming relationships, as well as preparing them for the changes to come. Including parents in the transition process enables their knowledge of their child's unique characteristics and early experiences to be included in the overall provision for transition: in Dockett and Perry's (2005a) work with ethnic minority parents in Australia, it was the parents themselves who identified the kind of support that would help their child with starting school, such as the provision of a network which would help them to make friends.

The argument that children's transitions must be understood as *family* transitions is not simply an acknowledgement of the difficulties that parents themselves may experience as they become 'parents of school pupils' rather than parents of pre-school children. A high-quality pre-school programme will have worked closely with the parents of the pre-school child in the child's care and education, and shared its goals and objectives for children – including the qualities which build resilience – with home care givers. Starting school may be a moment when the child is particularly vulnerable, and is definitely not the time to abandon parental partnerships, which are now more important than at any time since the child's first transition into group care.

Changing structures: moving towards continuity

The differences of perspective and practice described in the previous section arise, it is clear, from beliefs about children and childhood which have been 'set in stone' by the statutory arrangements made for children in the last hundred years and more. 'School starts at 5? Well then, that must be the appropriate age for children to get on with their learning . . .'. But there are now signs that policy-makers are responding to research evidence about children's transitions, and rethinking some of these enshrined beliefs and practices. As a result, some governments have begun to blur the boundaries between age-phases, and create more continuity from early into middle childhood.

Moving towards continuity in the UK

The recent devolution of power to national governments within the UK means that few new initiatives apply to all the nations in the Union, yet each is in its own way moving towards greater continuity for children. In England, the framework for the *Early Years Foundation Stage* (DfES 2007), has not only linked together provision for under-3s and over-3s, which previously operated under different sets of guidance and regulations. It has also integrated the National Care Standards, which previously applied to those settings which were viewed as non-educational, into the same set of guidelines, so that all those working with children from birth to 5 are required to share their expectations for children, based on a holistic view of development and an activity-based view of learning. For the first time, professionals with backgrounds in health and social care, as well as education, are required to think collaboratively about the opportunities they offer to children from birth into formal schooling.

In Wales, the Welsh Assembly pre-empted this move in 2003 with the planned introduction of a new education policy, *The Learning Country*, which was to include a Foundation Phase of education for all children aged from 3 to 7 (Welsh Assembly Government 2003). The new framework was piloted in 41 pre-school settings the following year, and extended into some Year 1 and Year 2 classrooms in 2005 (Siraj-Blatchford et al. 2006). The full implementation of the project is intended to ensure that by 2010 all Welsh children should be offered a seamless curriculum experience, from their entry into an education setting at 3, until their transfer into the later primary years at 7+. A similar though less structurally radical initiative in Scotland is currently extending early years' curriculum and pedagogy into Primary 1 and beyond, with a national *Curriculum for Excellence* planned for all children from 3 to 18 years (Carmichael and Hancock 2007), while a new 'Enriched Curriculum' has blurred the boundaries for many children in Northern Ireland (Walsh 2007) .

Every Child Matters

Discontinuity between services and providers, as well as between educational age-phases, has haunted successive UK governments, notably through a sequence of child abuse cases which subsequent inquiries have revealed to be the result of a failure to provide continuity of care for children. In 2003, after the judicial inquiry into one such case, the government published proposals for a comprehensive system of holistic care for all children, including the most vulnerable (Laming 2003).

This framework, *Every Child Matters* (DfES 2003), has been the blueprint for reorganizing and expanding services with the intention of offering all-day care and education to all children whose parents require it, from birth to the age of 14. Like the under-fives' framework, *Every Child Matters* has drawn on policies from New Zealand in framing broad areas of development and well-being as its goals. The goals for children, to which all services and practitioners are committed, are: staying safe, being healthy, enjoying and achieving, making a positive contribution, and achieving economic well-being. The numerous separate mechanisms and initiatives which are needed to implement such a broad-based policy are being put into place through new legislation and new funding. One of the earliest initiatives is the creation of 3500 children's centres – one for every community – charged with providing care and education for children under 5, a range of services for parents, opportunities for training and employment, and all the health, mental health and advice services that the particular community needs. One consequence of the children's centre initiative should be that many of the discontinuities which young children previously experienced are replaced by some continuity of care and care givers, as well as of curriculum and location. If the children's centre programme 'delivers', the transitions of children from birth to 5 may be smoother and happier than they have been, although the move into formal learning still awaits them.

Curriculum continuity: New Zealand

The early years curriculum developed in New Zealand during the 1990s has attracted admiration from around the world, and has influenced the design of subsequent initiatives in England. The framework, called *Te Whaariki*, or 'the woven mat', was based on the traditional ideas of children's development of the indigenous Maori people, and was intended to reflect the equal rights of all segments of the population to experience culturally appropriate environments and opportunities in their early childhood environments (NZ Ministry of Education 1996). The curriculum is grounded in five behavioural dispositions, which can be observed through close attention to children's activity in their settings: well-being (*mana atua*), belonging (*mana whenua*), contributing (*mana tangata*), communicating (*mana reo*) and exploring (*mana aoturoa*). In this holistic view of the child, it is understood that 'the main achievement occurs in the development of the child's *mana* ... Having *mana* is the enabling and empowering tool to controlling their own destiny' (Reedy 2003, cited by Peters 2007). Although there is said to be no equivalent in English for the term *mana*, it creates a vision of a child who is strong, empowered, and 'ready' to learn.

As with all innovative pre-school curricula, the obvious question was: what happens when children go to school and experience a formal, subject-based curriculum? In 2006, the government announced that a new primary curriculum based on 'key competencies' was to be launched, allowing similar qualities and dispositions to be prioritized. The document affirms that these competencies develop 'in social contexts' and 'over time, shaped by interactions with people, places and things'. Like other dispositions, they can not be taught but are fostered by the ethos of the environment.

Policy makers engaged in finalizing the plans for the new school-age curriculum are asking the question, 'what kinds of learners do we value in the 21st century?' (Peters 2007). This open-minded questioning seems a far cry from the subject-driven curricula of many other 'western democracies', and offers clear possibilities for continuity of experience – both curriculum and pedagogy – for children now entering the education system.

Transition programmes: stepping up through the school system

The last ten years have witnessed a huge increase in initiatives by school districts and education authorities to facilitate the progression from pre-school into the Reception or pre-primary year, and from this year into formal schooling. Both Harry and Louis, whose stories were presented earlier, benefited from such efforts. There is space here to mention just three of the many projects undertaken to support children's moves within the education system.

From pre-school to school: Norfolk SEN Transition support

This initiative in a largely rural area, with a wide range of different types of pre-school provision, was designed to give appropriate transition support to the children within the pre-school system who were already identified as having additional needs. Harry, described earlier, was one of its beneficiaries, but Norfolk Children's Services has developed a framework intended to enable all children with special needs to receive an equivalent level of support.

The transition programme commences at least half a year before children are due to move into mainstream school, with the completion of a child profile in which the child's current needs (medical, dietary, social and so on) are detailed, along with their strengths and difficulties in all areas of learning and behaviour. The child and parents, as well as the pre-school staff, contribute to this profile, which forms the basis for a Transition Plan. The plan involves all those who will be present during the transition period – from teachers, parents and support workers to the child's friends, and the driver who will escort the child to school. It includes arrangements for 'training', formal or informal, for all these important individuals, who will each have a role to play in supporting the child in the new setting. It also identifies the key resources which will help the child (visits, maps, videos, farewell activities, photo albums) and clear principles which everyone involved must observe. The last of these 'principles' could stand as a principle for all children's transitions, everywhere: 'Transition systems have to work for every child – if they do not, it is our problem, not the child's problem' (Norfolk Children's Services 2006). This locally based intervention aims to ensure that all children are offered the resources they need for transitions within the system.

From pre-primary to Primary 1: Northern Ireland

In Dungannon, County Tyrone, the early years' team at the Southern Education & Libraries Board (SELB) undertook a major transitions project in 2005. Staff visiting schools and settings had become conscious of the huge gulf in practice that existed between children's experiences in their Nursery classes and in Primary 1 (the first year of statutory school), even when the two classrooms were only yards apart. Funding was obtained for Nursery and Primary 1 teachers from 20 schools to spend time visiting their counterparts, and to attend seminars and discussions in which to compare and reflect on their practice. Participants were helped to undertake a series of classroom observations, which became the basis for discussion, and to identify the roles and competences of the children in each age-phase. Overwhelmingly, they reported that Nursery children were observed to behave more independently, and take on more responsibility, than children in Primary 1: as one P1 teacher told me, with surprise, 'The children sweep up the sand themselves – they do! And I've always done it for them'.

This experience of crossing borders, within a traditionally highly segmented system, brought new insights to all the participants and paved the way for changes in practice, in which many of the early years' teachers' beliefs and practices were carried forward into the start of primary school.

From Foundation Stage to Year 1: the Oxford Transitions Project

The Oxford Project, like many others, arose from 'a growing tide of feeling from teachers, children and parents, that children's experiences at the start of Year 1 were often discontinuous from those now embedded in the Foundation Stage' (Oxfordshire CC 2006: 2). Advisers in the county were conscious that the competences children demonstrated in their nursery classes appeared to vanish when they started formal schooling, and initiated a collaborative project involving teachers, headteachers, governors, advisers and consultants across the age range from 3 to 7. They looked at generic issues of discontinuity, and at the particular cases of more vulnerable children: those with special needs, or with English as an additional language, or those – such as refugee children and looked-after children – whose lives lacked a stable social and emotional base from which to 'move on'.

The 20 schools selected for the initiative undertook individual projects addressing concerns such as outdoor learning, role play and parent participation, each of which was written up for publication. The participants in every setting began by asking children to 'show us how you feel' about the move into Year 1, and took the children's expressed views – of happiness and excitement, sadness and fear – into account as they planned their actions. Each case study identifies 'what we have learnt' and reports realistically on the constraints that were experienced.

The larger group also worked towards general Principles for Transition, and produced an exemplary School Transition Plan as a model for other schools and settings to build on. Publication of the findings has enabled this limited project to be extended into all settings, for the support of all children.

Routes to continuity

Research on transitions over the last decade has clarified and verified a great deal of what we have always suspected, and argued, as practitioners in early years' settings. The discontinuities and difficulties we have all observed as young children are moved to larger, more complex institutions, and required to learn in more formal and more abstract ways, are replicated around the world, almost everywhere that children go to school.

Paradoxically, according to John Bennett (2006: 16), the only countries where such difficulties are not experienced are those which lack the kind of play-based early provision which most of us regard as desirable and appropriate for young children:

> In countries adopting a pre-primary approach to early education – that is, organising early education not as a kindergarten (with a focus on play, socio-emotional development, and holistic project work) but like a junior school (age cohorts, high child-staff ratios, a focus on cognitive development and learning standards, very few parental inputs) – transition into school is normally not a difficulty.

Bennett (2006: 16) goes on, however, to point out that this 'solution' to transition difficulties is not in children's best interests:

> One has the impression in this situation that the young children have never really had the experience of an appropriate early childhood pedagogy where they can learn self-regulation at their own pace and follow their own learning paths. The similarity of the two milieus supports a smooth transition from pre-primary into primary, but not necessarily at a personal level.

Evidently, the solution to transition difficulties does not lie down this particular path. Instead it relies on a two-fold approach:

- First, adults work together actively to reduce the discontinuities between phases.
- Second, pre-school children are helped to acquire the resources and resilience that will enable them to make 'good' transitions from phase to phase.

The individual case studies and the local initiatives described in this chapter could be replicated many times over, as educators and parents increasingly demonstrate their willingness to work together for children's well-being as they 'step up' through the system. The next chapter presents the children's own account of the experience, and what it means to them.

5

Children's perspectives:
transitions around the world

First I stayed in a playground, then in a childcare institution, now I am in kindergarten and then I will go to school and then to work, and then I will stop working and I will be free all day because I am growing old – Hans, age 6, Norway.

(Eide and Winger 1995, cited in Eide and Winger 2005: 71)

Listening to young children requires of adults some revaluing and relearning of other languages, which takes time and effort and presupposes a willingness to be multilingual. It is, in short, difficult for those who by adulthood have lost many of the hundred languages of childhood.

(Moss et al. 2005: 5)

It is hard to believe that, only a few short years ago, the idea of listening to children's own views on their lives, and on the arrangements made for them by adults, was deeply suspect. Young children were regarded as 'immature' and 'unreliable' beings, who had difficulty distinguishing fact from fiction and who certainly could not be trusted to have a say in important decisions about their own lives. All this has changed, as new constructions of the child as a meaning-maker, and as an active contributor to her own and others' lives, have been supported by a growing awareness of children's rights and their moral status in our society (Mayall 2002). 'Listening to children' is now recognized as a key responsibility for everyone involved in caring for or providing for young children, and such consultation is increasingly becoming mandatory in the evaluation and regulation of services and policies.

Children's own reports of their experiences in pre-schools and schools, and of the impact of transitions on their happiness and well-being, can contribute enormously to improving practice in schools and settings, informing policy-making, and guiding research agendas. As evidence accumulates from children around the world, it becomes clear that, despite regional and national and global variations, there are some key experiences and values that are important to children wherever they live, and go to school. This chapter asks what we can learn from listening to children's own views on their early transitions, and their own responses to the arrangements made for them. It begins with a brief account of the way that children's rights have been recognized in the last two decades, and of the current status of children's participation, before looking at the ways of 'listening' that have evolved during this period, and at what children have to say about what matters in their lives.

The right to a voice

The United Nations Convention on the Rights of the Child (UN 1989) which has been signed and ratified by almost every nation, provides a reference point for governments and non-governmental organizations as they set in place arrangements for children's lives. The complex provisions of the convention are often described as guaranteeing three key rights for children: protection, provision and participation (Alderson 2000). Protection, which ensures the survival, development and security of the child, can be guaranteed where adequate legislation and funding are available, and is provided to an acceptable level in most western societies and in some developing nations. Provision – of services such as health, education and cultural activities – is similarly secured through legislation and financial arrangements, and is offered at varying but generally adequate levels in the advanced industrial nations. Participation – the child's right to be informed, to be heard, and to be involved in decision-making – is much more difficult to legislate and monitor, and depends on a commitment by the adults who work with children, as well as by government and policy makers.

Children's participation rights are enshrined in Article 12 of the original convention, which requires signatories to 'Assure to the child who is capable of forming his or her own views the right to express those views freely in all matters affecting the child, the views of the child being given due weight in accordance with the age and maturity of the child'. Article 13 follows this up with a requirement that the child shall 'be provided the opportunity to be heard' in proceedings affecting the child.

The convention, however, can be seen to bestow rights with one hand, and simultaneously take them away with the other, since it leaves open the question of whether a child is 'capable of forming his or her own views', and whether the 'age and maturity of the child' require adults to listen to those views. It is left to the subjective belief of those implementing the convention to decide whether a child of, say, 3 or 4 years, is mature enough to hold views which adults should listen to. This is why the convention in itself can not safeguard children's participation rights, *unless* those who implement it view young children as competent and capable experts in their own lives.

Concerns over the wording of the convention, which caused some signatories to treat 'the child' as someone over the age of 12, prompted a further discussion in 2004 on 'Implementing child rights in early childhood' and the publication in 2005 of 'General Comment 7' arising from this discussion. The 'comment' affirms

> that young children are holders of all rights enshrined in the convention, and that early childhood is a critical period for the realization of these rights. The Committee's working definition of 'early childhood' is all young children: at birth and throughout infancy; during the pre-school years; as well as during the transition to school.
>
> (CRC 2005: 1)

In relation to Article 12, it points out that, 'in many countries and regions', traditional beliefs have constructed children as 'undeveloped, lacking even the basic capacities for understanding, communicating and making choices' (CRC 2005: 7). These beliefs are contradicted by the assurance that

> article 12 applies both to younger and to older children. As holders of rights, even the youngest children are entitled to express their views ... They make choices and communicate their feelings, ideas and wishes in numerous ways, long before they are able to communicate through the conventions of spoken or written language.
>
> (CRC 2005: 7)

Finally, the Comment points out that, for this right to be assured, adults would need to 'adopt a child-centred attitude, listening to young children and respecting their dignity and their individual points of view'. Furthermore, they would need to show 'patience and creativity' as they learned to adapt to children's 'preferred ways of communicating'. The agenda for children's participation is thus very explicitly set out, and applies to all parents, providers, practitioners, and of course to researchers.

Researching children's perspectives with 'patience and creativity'

Observing newborn babies

As the CRC Comment recognizes, children find ways to express their feelings and preferences about their care long before they acquire language (and many babies would not survive without this facility). Researchers have only recently paid much attention to these feelings, however. One very striking example is the work in neonatal units of Alderson et al. (2005), whose close observations of the 'signs' given out by very small premature babies in their early days of life, often in intensive care, reveals very distinct preferences for certain types of care, by certain types of people. Even before they were technically 'mature' enough to be born, these tiny infants could demonstrate their awareness of who was handling them, and how, and of the levels of light, noise and activity around them. They could communicate, to an attentive observer, their reactions to their very abrupt transition into a world for which they were not fully prepared, and the conditions which helped to support and comfort them through the experience. As with any other transition, close attention to the experiences of these children not only assured sensitive care for them, but also enabled recommendations to be made for the care of babies faced with similar experiences.

Using the MOSAIC approach with toddlers

As they gain in mobility, agility and expressive skills, children under 3 in group-care settings are able to offer a wealth of information to the 'patient and creative' listener, and their communicative competence has been demonstrated very clearly through the development of the MOSAIC approach (Clark and Moss 2001). Clark and Moss drew upon all the information that was available to researchers, practitioners and parents of a sample of young children in one nursery, and used it to piece together a picture of the children's own likes and dislikes. The 'mosaic' included observations of the child – made by the researcher and the child's key worker, and discussed between them and the parents; interviews with parents to elicit their view of their child's preferences; and participatory data from the children: photographs taken with disposable cameras, or video clips of a tour of the nursery in which the child led the researcher around and pointed out important people, places and activities. Where possible, the child's friends or older siblings also contributed information, or accompanied the child on the 'tour', or handled the video camera. Individual children are involved in sorting and displaying the photographs, or commenting on the video, or making their own drawings and maps of the nursery. They acquire the skills to review their earlier pictures, and talk about the adults and places, friends and activities, that are important to them.

As with the newborns, these children's strong feelings about their nursery day can both inform their current care, and their move into the next setting, and help staff to plan for the next generation of children who will come into the nursery, and move through different areas in the years before school.

Listening to the languages of pre-school children

Participatory methods, such as playing games, taking pictures, drawing and storytelling, offer a range of ways for practitioners and researchers to listen to children's 'hundred languages', and gain greater insights into children's perspectives on their pre-school settings. With older pre-school children, and the youngest schoolchildren, Alison Clark (2005) has expanded the MOSAIC activities into extended projects on map making and book making, in which individual children's voices are combined in group projects which build on their skills in making meaning and co-constructing knowledge. This more interactive approach is based on a belief that 'listening' does not mean simply 'finding out what is already in children's heads' rather it is an activity which supports children in exploring and sharing ideas, attaining new perspectives and arriving at fresh conclusions.

In order to support children's meaning-making in this way, the adult researcher has to dispel children's common belief that adults who ask questions (especially adults in schools and pre-schools) nearly always know the answers, and are actually just testing children on their knowledge. Instead, children need to feel that they are being recognized as the experts in this particular field, and have the power and knowledge to share their expertise if they so choose. This reversal of the usual adult–child power relation is achieved in different ways: sometimes simply by the adult's honest assurance, and the children's trust in this assurance; sometimes by asking children to answer questions posed by a puppet or soft toy; often, by asking them to think what information and advice they would give to a new child just starting in the setting. Siting the 'conversations' in locations of the children's choice – in the garden or home corner or block area – enables them to show the adult what they do, and even include the adult in their play (Clark 2005). In this situation, children are able to disagree with each other, or modify other children's comments, without risk of giving the 'wrong' answer. The results of such conversations can surprise us.

School views: using children's talents

As children proceed into formal schooling, their range of communicative competencies becomes seemingly infinite. So long as they are assured that their own knowledge is genuinely valued and appreciated, they become endlessly helpful in explaining and illustrating their point of view, enjoying group discussions and paired interviews, role plays and board games, drawing and map making, completing child-friendly tasks and questionnaires, and collecting dossiers of information and evidence to present and discuss. School-age children can be forthright in their views, and often enjoy the status of a formal interview, in which their words are recorded verbatim and quoted back to them (Brooker 2001). In busy classrooms there may not be many opportunities for children to air personal opinions, so the chance to be consulted formally on their likes and dislikes, preferences and prejudices, may help them to organize and manage their own responses to the institutional requirements they face. Communicating their views can be empowering for children so long as they are confident they are being listened to by adults who are also willing, in Warming's (2005: 53) term, to 'make common cause with the children'.

What do children tell us about their transitions?

The evidence of children's own views in the following sections derives from a range of published and unpublished sources, and I am grateful to everyone in the wider network of 'transitions' researchers who has sent me their own transcripts and stories. (See the Acknowledgements for further details.)

Children under 3

As Chapter 2 suggested, few studies have been made of the preferences of very young children as they enter their first day-care settings. Nevertheless children's feelings are very evident to an alert observer, and these in-depth studies show how much can be achieved when parents and practitioners – and researchers – collaborate closely to identify them. Pre-verbal children, or those like Yuk-Yue with limited language, tell their parents and key workers how they feel about attending nursery in many ways: both Yuk-Yue's mother and her key worker Kerry had identified as significant the moment every day when the little girl stopped outside the door, as if holding her breath in anticipation, then smiled, 'sang a song' and ran in.

Case studies of such early transitions – including studies in New Zealand (Dalli 2002), Denmark (Thyssen 2000) and the USA (Daniel and Shapiro 1996) – can reveal the aspects of children's experience which contribute to their well-being and belonging. All of these observations show children actively constructing pleasurable experiences for themselves through their interactions with children, adults, objects and the environment.

Early friendships

In Thyssen's (2000) study, as among the City Fields toddlers, spontaneous displays of physical affection between 'new' children and others in the setting indicate the enormous pleasure that sociable young children gain from simply being together. Thyssen's description of Sarah's behaviour with her peers was very reminiscent of Hana's relationship with Billy (see Chapter 2), but he points out that reciprocity takes time to become established, and that children's early 'communications' may be through involvement in shared activities, or through using objects to communicate. Adults, he argues, must therefore watch and participate in shared activities, and actively consider 'how it is possible to support the children's first orientation towards each other and their starting a common life' (2000: 45).

Objects and activities

Observations of the children at City Fields confirmed the views of parents and care givers that the environment and activities offered by the setting were key to children's successful transitions and their sense of well-being. Children became deeply involved, for instance, in solitary play with sand, with home-corner resources, and with trucks and cars that could be 'vroomed' along surfaces and trundled through vegetation. At such times they often talked or sang to themselves, or to their doll or truck, and showed their total sense of security and well-being by their relaxed limbs and facial expressions, as well as their secret smiles and giggles. Children with limited indoor and outdoor space at home revelled in the freedom and opportunities provided by their new setting.

As Clark's (2001, 2005) studies confirm, many of the spaces and resources in nurseries hold very special meanings for young children, and assure them of the safety and security of their world.

Relating to adults
Children's proactive efforts to establish relationships with their key workers and other staff are also widely observed. Thyssen describes a child aged 14 months, in her second week in day care, who initiates brief affectionate encounters with three different practitioners within a short period of time, *not*, as he reports, because she needs to be comforted; rather, 'it takes place in a joyful mood' (2000: 41). Dalli's observations of children's preferences for particular care givers mirror those in the Danish settings, but also reflect the type of child–care giver relationship that the centre promotes. Dalli comments on 'the consistency with which the patterns of interactions that children established with the centre adults fitted with the centre's policies and the teachers' expectations for how this pattern would unfold' (2000:4). Although this comment suggests some constraints on children's options, all of the case study children found ways to forge the relationships that suited them with the adults of their choice, despite centre policies which could have prevented this.

At City Fields too, as the case studies in Chapter 2 demonstrated, children quickly showed their new care givers the type of relationship that suited their personal needs, and the watchful adults responded accordingly. As they grew in confidence, many children still relied on their key worker for comfort at the start of the day, or when they were hurt or upset; they checked that they were still around, and visible, at occasional moments; and they engaged them as play partners when they felt the need. The high levels of well-being shown by children in these settings compare dramatically with observations of children in poorer settings, and emphasize that adults must 'listen' with all their senses to discover what kinds of resource the children wish them to be.

Moving from pre-school to school

As Chapter 4 has shown, the 'discontinuities' between children's experiences of pre-school and school may outweigh the discontinuities they have experienced in their first move into group care. Children's own accounts of the transition reveal a great deal of resilience, but few suggest that the process was smooth or painless. The children's voices reported in this section are from countries as different as Bangladesh and China, Fiji and Guyana, but they share a common viewpoint.

Memories of pre-school
Children recall similar 'favourite' activities, almost everywhere. These children, aged between 5 and 7, had all moved on to primary school:

> We had activities like swinging and sliding, playing with sand, household corner, shop corner, carpentry corner and story telling from our teachers or from some of the mothers who come and help the teachers.
>
> (Fiji)

> You go to nursery school, and eat, and nursery school teaches you about Jesus, and for children to play with you and you can't fight. You have to play all the time.
>
> (Guyana)

> There were these things you could ride on, and you could climb up on and you could slide down on, and you could play on. We had a gate that we could come in at, and that was really fun.
>
> (Ireland)

> They had a home corner, a playground, games, cars and only one table to play games.
>
> (Portugal)

Only in Nigeria, which has a pre-primary rather than an early childhood tradition, were children unable to recall a play-based experience: 'While in pre-primary we study English and mathematics and learn to read. We are still doing that' (Nigeria). Even in this system however, children identify a different attitude and demeanour in their teachers. This is one of the commonest and saddest themes to emerge from the children surveyed in ten countries.

The changing face of teachers
Although some children report rumours of teachers beating and caning children which the researchers (such as O'Kane 2007) are careful to contradict, others evidently attend primary schools where the fear of physical or verbal violence was real:

> In this school I have to sit like this [indicates rows] and facing the teacher and do work on the blackboard whether you like it or not. This is no good. You answer wrongly you get scolded by the teacher. Most of the time I keep quiet. I fear getting scolded and a dong on my head.
>
> (Fiji)

Of the two *Apas* in my present school, one sometimes scolds us but never hits us. The other isn't at all pretty: she's dark and hits us whole time. She hits us whether we learn our lessons or not, sometimes for no reason. The *Apa* in the pre-school never hit us.

(Bangladesh)

The teachers are stricter. Sometimes I'm afraid of them. I'm afraid of Miss Hu the most, she is in charge of our class and teaches us Chinese.

(China)

In Portugal too, the primary school teachers were felt to be less sympathetic. Even if the children exaggerate, their comparisons between preschool and primary teachers reflect a real experience: 'at primary they shout', 'here the Head took away the ball', 'here sometimes they hit us'. It appears that the different background, training and ethos of pre-school and primary teachers afford very different relationships with their pupils.

No more play
One universal aspect of children's move to statutory schooling seems to be the loss of opportunities for play. The Irish children in O'Kane and Hayes's (2007) study report with some sadness that they are now only allowed to play on Friday, but like all the children they accept that this is an inevitable consequence of becoming a school pupil. The Portuguese children seem proud to report that

At pre-school we only played – at primary we study!

We spent all the afternoon at the carpet, we hardly did anything. At primary I work and sometimes we learn letters.

At pre-school we played! I didn't learn sums, reading, or any work … here, yes.

The Chinese and Nigerian children took a similar pride in their accomplishments:

If you don't go to school you cannot know more words. You only learn simple words at pre-school. If you don't go to school, you cannot learn more difficult knowledge.

(China)

I feel happy to be in school especially when I am given work and I am able to complete it and when I learn new things like computer.

(Nigeria)

In the Valley School (Brooker 1996) I followed a group of children from their last term in a nursery class through to the end of their Reception year, and found that pre-school children who were about to transfer into 'big school' had an exaggerated awareness of the differences and difficulties to come. One child who was interviewed offered a concise account of the changes that she thought would be required of her, but affirmed her own willingness to leave behind the activities she enjoyed, in order to be a good pupil. Cassie described both her favourite activities (painting, water, playing) and the problems she anticipated with school work. She assured me that she was ready to embark on 'work' in general, 'reading' (which she described as 'easy ... or a bit hard'), writing (which in order to be 'proper' must always be 'little') and 'numbers' (some of which she admitted were 'difficult'). In conclusion she volunteered the following assurance: 'I've got good news for you: when I come in your big class I am going to *do what you say!* When I go in your big class I am going to be quiet for you, not shout!'. Like all the children in this cohort, Cassie expected to give up the activities she enjoyed most, and adopt more restrained behaviour, when she started school. But she accepted that this was an inevitable part of the process, and showed neither reluctance nor resistance.

Being a pupil: adapting to the system

Dockett and Perry's (2002, 2004, 2005a, 2005b) longitudinal *Starting School* study in Australia confirms the findings from smaller studies, which identify children's concern with rules and taboos, their expectation of academic learning or 'hard work', and their acceptance of their own status as relatively powerless individuals within a hierarchical system

Keeping the rules
Many of children's concerns centre on the importance of learning the 'rules of school' rather than on the problems associated with academic work. Children everywhere quickly learn what kinds of behaviour are permitted in school, and can discuss with confidence the kinds of knowledge a new pupil would need.

Getting this information right is clearly an integral part of a successful transition. The Chinese children report that only 10 minutes of play is allowed every day, and explain the system which requires them to clean their own classroom, with a subsequent loudspeaker announcement to say which classrooms are cleanest: 'It will be broadcasted whether it is clean or not, such as Class One, Grade One; Class Two, Grade One'. The Irish children have a catalogue of information to impart to a new pupil:

about standing in line when the bell goes, about asking for the toilet (preferably in Irish), and about avoiding the major crimes of kicking, throwing books, throwing food, 'shouting out' rather than putting your hand up, and 'being bold':

[Child]   When you are in big school and you are bold, you will be sent to Mr Delaney...

[Researcher] *And what would you do to be bold? What is bold?*

[Child]   Well, Ruairi is really bold. He bited someone's finger yesterday...

[Pause]

[Child]   Mr Delaney said if anyone was bold he would just bring them to his office ... and every day for nine days he would give them a slap, because they would be bold.

These children, a matter of weeks after starting school are confident rather than cowed, and find strength in solidarity. But despite their sparky resilience, it is clear that they are accepting the presence and persistence of a power relationship which does not work in their favour. As Dockett et al. (2002: 350) affirm,

Children are particularly keen to adjust to school. They want to know the rules and they are aware of issues related to power; for example, they know that teachers make the rules for the class, and that school principals make rules for teachers.

All the children consulted in this Australian project display a concern with the rules and taboos of classrooms, and the consequences of infringing them: 'children were adamant that they needed to know the school rules in order to function well within the school and, in particular, to keep out of trouble' (Dockett and Perry 2002: 80). They confidently generated long lists of forbidden behaviours, some common to schools everywhere ('Don't run', 'You're not allowed to hit', 'No kicking') but some specific to a particular setting or classroom:

Have to line up at the dots
Can't touch the piano
Stay in your own proper chair
Know to sit down or stand up if the teacher says
Not allowed to run away.

(Dockett and Perry 2002: 80)

In common with the Irish children, they feared being sent to the principal, as well as reckoning with the lesser punishments of 'time out' or having their names written up on a board. In one class, 'the shock of "getting your name on the board" and then not knowing how to get it off, caused considerable anxiety for a group of new school children' (Dockett and Perry 2007: 100).

These authors point out that a change in the ways that discipline is enforced, and good behaviour promoted, is one of the major discontinuities for children. In pre-school settings, unacceptable behaviours are usually discussed with the child and group with some gentleness and understanding, whereas in school there may be summary punishments. Similarly, the warm praise and personal acknowledgement which results from 'good' behaviour in pre-schools may be rewarded in school by more extrinsic means such as star charts and merit cards. Children show an awareness of these differences, which they have picked up from older friends and siblings, and from the media, well before they start school. Einarsdottir (2007: 80), reviewing international studies, reports that in many societies 'the children seemed to have internalized a traditional and stereotypical view of school ... they seemed to take the rules for granted and did not question them'.

Hard work
The stereotype of school life as 'hard work' is one promoted by parents as well as older children, and is viewed with equal measures of pride and reluctance by children in the early months of school. Studies in the Nordic countries, cited by Einarsdottir (2007) confirm that children believe it is right and proper to work hard in school, just as it was right and proper to play in pre-school. To some extent they would be disappointed if this promise failed to materialize: in a Swedish study, the children 'believed that the elementary school stands for the right way of learning and that pre-school was training for elementary school' (Einarsdottir 2007: 79). Similar views were expressed by children in other European countries, many of whom characterized the different experience of formal schooling in terms of 'sitting at desks', 'sitting in rows' or 'facing the front', just like the Fijian child quoted earlier.

The Irish children interviewed by O'Kane seem unsure whether they should profess to love their school work, or hate it, but their group interviews allow them to try out different perspectives, as the following extract shows (O'Kane and Hayes 2007: np):

[Researcher] If you could choose one thing to do more of what would that be?
[Child 1] I'd do loads and loads and loads more work. And I'd do exams, and I'd do pluses, and reading ...

[Researcher] Wow, lots more work, what do the rest of you think?
[Child 2] I'd do the same.
[Child 1] We love our workbooks don't we?
[Child 3] I hate it.
[Child 4] So do I. I hate every book except maths. I hate school.
[Child 3] Except Fridays.
[Child 5] I like Fridays.

Friday, of course, is the only day when they are allowed to play.

Children involved in the Oxfordshire Transitions project (described in Chapter 4) showed a similar mix of fears and enthusiasm as they moved into the first year of a statutory curriculum. Asked to draw themselves and dictate captions in response to the instruction, 'Show us how you feel', some described their pleasure at the prospect of doing 'difficult spellings' or more serious computer work, and one drew himself smiling broadly as he looked forward to 'a reading book with harder words'. Others however described themselves as 'worried': 'I'm a little bit worried about the work. We'll have to do hard work'; 'I'm worried at going to school because I don't like doing writing because I can't do it'; another wrote simply, 'Do you have to do hard things?' (Oxfordshire CC 2006).

A *new identity*

Cassie, interviewed in the Valley School, was confident of her ability both to assume a new 'pupil' identity, and to be as competent in her new roles and responsibilities as in the ones she exercised in nursery. For other children however, the task of taking on a new identity inspires considerable fear and anxiety, and the major identity shift of 'becoming a school pupil' offers many potential hazards. Children's sense of self is formed through the relationships they experience with others, from birth and then in successive new environments. A child whose identity is secure and comfortable in her home may feel insecure and uncomfortable when the demands made on her change, and entry to school may be an occasion when she feels less supported, and less competent, than during earlier transitions. The 'hard work' and rules of behaviour offer specific challenges to the child's self-esteem, as we have seen, but other aspects of identity may also be at stake. Even the most confident child will need the reassurance that other children, and unfamiliar adults, find them acceptable in the new setting.

The Oxfordshire project enabled participating children to voice some of their doubts about the ways they would be viewed and treated by others, and their ability to conform to expectations. While the 'hard work' anxieties centred on the new classroom and teacher, children's sense of self was also at risk in the playground:

> I'm not looking forward to the big playground, there might be people I don't know ...
> I'm not happy if no-one plays with me ...
> I'm afraid of the big children ... the older children might be horrible ...

One child pleaded, 'I want the older kids to know, "Do not bully" '. The brief period when children are unsure whether they will lose their existing friends, and fear that they may not make new friends, is one in which they need sensitive support from adults. Children who know their friends will accompany them, by contrast, name this as the main reason for looking forward to their new class.

The loss of confidence is understood by other children as a reason why it is not unusual to cry. The Irish children in O'Kane's (2007) groups discussed this occurrence with some enthusiasm, offering explanations on behalf of other children ('she wanted to stay with her mam') and on their own: 'It was a bit scary, I was a bit scared, because all adults were talking to me an all, and that was a bit scary'. Other children were recalled as scared of particular curriculum activities, and of particular adults. Reassuringly, these children assert confidently, even in their first weeks at school, that 'someone will tell the teacher' if a child is teased or crying in the school yard, and that teachers will sort the problem out.

Similar comments are made in the entirely different context of a small study in Brunei (Kitson 2004), where crying is viewed by children as well as parents as a natural response to starting school. Children who started school with a friend or sibling explained how important this was: 'I didn't cry, I was happy because I started with my cousin'; but it was assumed that those who started unaccompanied would be distressed, 'scared' and 'insecure' (Kitson 2004: 239). The children's own reports mirror those of the Oxford children:

> I was worried about starting because I was afraid of the teacher ...
> I was sad and unhappy on the first day and I cried ...
> I was sad about going to school and I was worried because I had no friends at school.

The author summarizes, 'Separating from their parents, not having friends and being afraid of the teacher were the reasons given by children for their negative feelings about starting school' (Kitson 2004: 240).

We may wonder, when children give us such clear signals, why we seem so reluctant to act on them. On the one hand, of course, we can argue that most children *are* resilient and *do* adapt to the new arrangements; and that experiencing stressful change itself contributes to resilience, and paves the way for future adaptations. On the other hand, we should ask ourselves whether current arrangements for transitions supply children with the resources they need to cope well; and whether the new environments children enter need to be quite so different from the familiar ones which they have learned to love. I will return to these questions.

'Why do children go to school?'

One important factor in children's sense of control over their own lives, particularly during transitions, is their belief that there is a real purpose, a 'good reason' for the move they are required to make. Even young children develop an understanding that there are cost-benefits in experiences they dislike, from taking medicine and having injections to queuing at a checkout or waiting for a train. Babies and toddlers cannot be expected to work out that their parents have to leave them in group care, but pre-school and school children can and do formulate their own explanations for attending a setting. Their reasons offer insights into their understanding of their place in the world – in relation to adults and institutions, and in relation to the present and the future. Understanding the purpose of transitions can enable children to approach them positively and to acquire resilience for future life events.

Children's explanations for their attendance at school or pre-school range along a continuum from compulsion to volition: from 'have to' to 'want to'. Children who emphasize the compulsive element offer a range of reasons why society makes such a requirement: as a result they may feel reluctant or resistant in the setting. Children who cite their own volition obviously approach their experiences with greater readiness and enthusiasm. But right across the continuum there reigns a sense that school is 'good for you', which helps a lot of children to develop reasonably positive attitudes to their moves through the education system.

'Because you have to'

Knowing that the arrangements made for you by adults are non-negotiable is not necessarily cause of negative feelings, but may discourage commitment and enthusiasm for learning. Children in the All Saints' study (Brooker 2002) included many such explanations in their accounts, suggesting that they could identify both societal requirements and the needs of their parents:

[Researcher] Why do you think children go to school?
[Callum]   Because you have to, just because you do, I just know you do.
[Kerry]   Because their mum's had enough of them staying at home – I told my mum I don't want to go to school and she said, you have to.

More than one child revealed how these requirements are enforced:

[Robbie]   If you don't the police will get you, if you miss school you got to go another day...

Some children can sympathize with their parents' point of view:

[Katie]   Because mums have to go and get their money from the post office.
[Rufia]   So they can go to sleep: mummy looking after two babies, she's tired!

The group of Fijian children referred to earlier could not suggest any positive reasons for being in school and clearly felt considerable reluctance to be there:

[Researcher] So, why do children go to school?
[Child 1]   Some of us children just go to school because our parents told us to do so!
[Child 2]   Children like me go to school because they have to and it is what the old people say.
[Child 3]   I don't know why children go to school – it's probably they have to.

Many children, reflecting the cultural expectations of their society, point out that starting school is age-related, and that therefore you start because you are 'big' rather than for any other reason. A Japanese girl explains, 'Because I became 4 years old I am here' whereas Sonia (from All Saints') explains, 'Because I ain't 4 no more, I'm 5 – I had a birthday and I got earrings!'

To work, to play ... and to behave

Some children's reasoning is rather circular on this matter in their first term at school, and they report on what they *do* at school as their reason for being there. At All Saints', most of the English-speaking children in the class additionally explained they went to school to play:

Just to play toys and sit on a seat and do drawing ...
To play with the sand and water ...
Play with sand and play with playdough ...
That's where you play and do puzzles.

Children from Bangladeshi families in the same class were more likely to report that they came to school to 'learn reading', 'learn writing' or simply to 'study'. These responses are echoed by children inter-nationally: 'to learn things and learn to read' (Ireland), 'to learn to read and write', 'to learn to be attentive, to read and to speak English' (Nigeria), 'to learn more words and difficult knowledge' (China).

In the Valley School study (Brooker 1996), pre-school children like Cassie gave confident and positive explanations of the necessity for learning, and for how this would be achieved. Roisin had an older sister who had explained: 'To learn our spelling tests and our 2-times table. You write down all the hard words ... mum and dad teach you the words, then you go to school and write them down for the teacher'. Almost all the children, including all of the girls in this group, gave similar answers, before and during their first year of school, although all gave 'playing' as another important reason. They were equally con-vinced, like children in other studies, that going to school means learning the rules of behaviour (the fact that you would not *need* to learn these rules if you were not at school does not occur to anyone). Some children go to school, it appears, to learn to tidy, to help tidy the classroom, and to eat all their dinner up; others, to hang their coats on the hook properly, to 'listen for your name' (in the register) and just 'to be good'.

[Khiernssa] They go to school because they want to be busy, because their teacher's going to say, Good boy, and Good girl. I know that because I am a good girl.

These children have assented to the school's moral ethos without apparent difficulty and, as Einarsdottir (2007) concludes, believe that they are in the right place and doing the right thing for children of their age.

Future goals

In some societies more than others, children's understanding of their transition into school seems strongly linked to future goals: some societies, for economic or political reasons, place a greater or more explicit emphasis on children's future contribution to the general good. Among the children whose views were recently sampled, those from China, Nigeria and Bangladesh showed the strongest commitment to their future role. A Nigerian girl explained, 'We go to school so that we can learn and help people. We can become lawyers or doctors and help our parents', while the Bangladeshi children had aspirations to be pre-school teachers, policemen and engineers (and in one instance, a gangster with a helicopter). These children all understood that going to school was a prerequisite for going to college and taking exams, while one 6-year-old Chinese boy had the whole sequence figured out: 'You finish the study at pre-school, if you don't go to school where can you go? First it's primary school, then middle school and high school. And you get a job and then you'll die – pass away. I mean, you'll become an old man'.

Most of the children who have been interviewed make some reference to the future, explaining that you need to go to school to learn to read, in order to get a job and earn money. But this long-term, future-oriented rationale offers less motivation for children than one which focuses on the experiences of the present: on the satisfaction of mastering the new knowledge and skills associated with 'being a pupil'.

What makes a 'good' transition?

It is not difficult to identify common themes from the evidence reported earlier, across the age range from infancy to school and across a range of national contexts. Despite developmental and cultural differences, children's needs during transitions are not dissimilar, and could be summarized as follows.

1 *A sense of self-worth and a positive sense of identity*: achieved through the experience of warm and supportive interactions during and after the transition; through acceptance of their vulnerability and anxieties, and comfort for their distress; through reassurance as to their competency and adequacy; and through acknowledgement of their considerable achievements in taking their first steps into a new environment.
2 *The presence of trusted and familiar adults*: the company of family members and familiar care givers from the former setting; gradual introductions to the new care givers; appropriate information and reassurance about those in charge of the new setting; well-trained and well-informed practitioners with a good understanding of children's developmental needs and of their rights.

3 *Friends and familiar peers*: ideally, the company of children from the former setting; where this is not possible, proactive work by practitioners to build children's social networks through key groups and activities; careful monitoring of children's ability to form relationships, support for their friendships and assistance with resolving conflicts.

4 *Understanding of rules and routines*: careful induction into all the important aspects of the school or setting; explicit but positive teaching about acceptable behaviours and the ways these are supported; clear reminders of transitions occurring within the day, and of the demands made by each of these; close monitoring and reinforcement for children who have difficulty grasping the requirements of the setting. (At the same time, a re-examination by adults of the reasons for all the rules of school may be called for.)

5 *A sense of control and purpose*: care and educational arrangements which allow children as many opportunities as possible to exercise choice, participate in decisions, care for their own physical needs and control the direction of their activities and learning; guidance in understanding emotions and feelings; support for positive dispositions and autonomous learning.

6 *An environment of opportunities*: activities and resources which enable children to participate at their own level, and support to extend their involvement in activities and their exploration of ideas and materials; time and space for individual and group interests to develop and flourish; opportunities for vigorous physical movement and outdoor experiences.

Children's voices show us that they fundamentally desire transitions; that they have no real wish to 'stay behind' in the nursery or pre-school once they have seen the challenges offered to children at the next stage; that they accept the constraints and even drudgery of some school learning because they see themselves as on a journey through the system; that they are keen to become more competent, to take more responsibility, to grow more like the adults they know and esteem. At the same time these voices suggest that if adults were to listen harder, they would provide more of the resources children require to make these transitions smoothly.

Listening to children

Listening to children's voices, as Hanne Warming (2005: 53) argues, may mean simply 'hearing and interpreting what you hear', or it may mean 'making a common cause with the children'. In relation to the evidence discussed in this chapter, we may either find out about children's perspectives, or try to act on their perspectives and on their behalf. Some of the themes to emerge from these voices are matters we can act on: making transitions less sudden and less scary in the ways I have suggested, and providing resources that will increase children's resilience and foster their reciprocity. Other themes, though, require us to search beneath their words for the messages they are communicating, and to recognize that those messages have come from us, the adults in society.

Public policies inevitably filter down to children as they hear their parents and other care givers talk; they will know, and accept, that investment in early years settings has many other objectives than just providing them with a place to be with friends, have fun and explore; that early childhood policies are also about enabling parents to work, preparing children for school, and supporting the social and economic goals of the community. So far, so good. But in the next phase of their education, we may feel that children's acceptance of the arrangements sometimes goes too far: that their expressed willingness to give up the (educational) activities they most enjoy, to lose control of their learning and even to submit to harsh or arbitrary discipline, in order to adapt to society's expectations, is too complicit. The Oxfordshire child who asks, 'Do you have to do hard things?' and his class mate who pleads, 'I want the older kids to know: Do not bully', along with all the children who cry on starting school, should be listened to; like the little child who announces that the Emperor has no clothes, they are asking questions that society should be asking of itself.

The fact, then, that children need and desire change, and feel positive and enthusiastic about new challenges and new learning, should not blind us to the evidence (Alderson 2002; Mayall 2002) that primary education, with its origins in the factory system, has a tendency to remove some of the rights that children have previously exercised, including the right to self-regulation, and the right to respect from others. In facilitating transitions, we should be wary of simply helping children to give up their rights without a protest. This requires us to enter a wider dialogue about the nature of our educational goals, and the ways we go about achieving them. This dialogue is outside the scope of this book, but points us again to the question: are schools ready for children?

6

Making the grade: the role of assessment in transitions

There were a lot of differences between pre-school and school ... We were all there in straight lines sitting and waiting what to be done. There was a lot of writing on the exercise books. There were to be no noises, we have to be quiet and whisper at all times. I think if children are to choose between going to pre-school and school, most of us would choose pre-school.

(School child, Fiji)

When children are listened to, the power balance tips towards the child. Assessment practice, however, implies that the adult has a pre-set agenda, in which case the power balance tips dramatically the other way – towards the adult.

(Carr et al. 2005: 129)

There may appear to be rather a large leap from listening to children's views on their transitions, to discussing assessment practices, but this chapter argues that there is no such leap, rather that we should view 'listening to children' as our main mode of assessment, particularly at times of transition. The key principle underpinning this argument is that 'listening' and 'assessing' share a common purpose: to give children control of their own learning, and enable them to manage the new environments they encounter, and the new challenges these environments set. This chapter suggests too that, at the point in children's transitions through the education system when we start to separate 'listening' from 'assessing', we are liable to jeopardize their continuing competence and confidence, so that the different modes of assessment that children encounter as they 'step up' through the system may be as disheartening for them as the other, more obvious, discontinuities we have already discussed.

So in this chapter I attempt to trace a path through the maze of assessment theory and practice, and to argue that the principles under-pinning child-centred, 'listening' assessments could be sustained through the transition from pre-school to the early years of formal schooling. The chapter considers the ways that adults typically assess young children – the *when* and *where*, *what* and *why* and *how* of assess-ment – and relates these to our current understandings of the way that knowledge and skills, dispositions and feelings are acquired and sus-tained when young children learn together in group settings.

In making the case for an understanding of 'learning' as a shared and social activity, and of 'assessment' as equally situated and con-textualized, I call on examples of good practice from around the world, and from decades of developing perspectives in this field. I ask, first and foremost:

- What do we want children to 'learn' in their early childhood settings?
- How can we use assessment to give children control of their learning?
- How can child-friendly assessment practices support children's transitions, as they move into the more abstract and formal learning environments of the middle years of schooling?

But first, my own 'learning story'.

Case study: learning self-assessment at the Valley School

The previous chapter described my own first experience, as a practi-tioner, of consulting children in nursery and reception classes. There is more to this story, and it has to do with my eyes being opened to chil-dren's competence at self-assessment. Chapter 5 described the interviews undertaken with children before and after their transition into my Reception class at the Valley School, and drew attention both to their awareness of the 'work ethic' that they presumed awaited them in school, and to their willingness to adopt this perspective as their own. My intention in talking to the children was to identify ways of sustaining the autonomy and independence they showed in the nursery, and to avoid socializing them too thoroughly into the compliant attitudes of school pupils. Before long, it became clear to me that assessment was both a key component of the children's expectations of school, and a key mechanism through which teachers controlled and regulated their behaviour, as well as their learning. In an effort to unseat these expectations (on the children's part) and regulatory tendencies (on my own) I introduced the children to the notion that they, rather than I, should assess their classroom learning.

With guidance from a short course I was attending, taught by Pat Gura (1996), the first steps I undertook were to withhold evaluative praise from children, and to listen to their own unprompted self-evaluations. The discipline of unlearning my own acquired habit of commenting approvingly and enthusiastically on children's efforts was the hardest step, but reading evidence from High/Scope trainers and other research sources (Green and Lepper 1974; Hitz and Driscoll 1988) did eventually persuade me that in praising children I was demonstrating my own ability to judge them and their performance just as surely as if I was criticizing them. The difficulty I experienced in accepting this rather obvious fact was matched by the puzzlement on the children's faces as I practised my neutral and non-committal responses to their work: not 'Wow! That's great, I love it!' but rather 'Ah ... you've finished your painting ... are you pleased with it?'

At the same time as withholding my own judgements, I learned to listen to the children's judgements – as often to themselves as to others – on their own efforts. The running commentaries children engaged in as they wrote and drew and looked at books gave me material to feed back to them when we started the more overt process of self-assessment:

Oops, I started at the wrong end...
Oh no, my line's all wonky...
Erm ... that doesn't really look like my nan, I think I'll have another go!
My 6s are better than Liam's 6s but my ones are bigger than his ones.

Before long the children learned that when they showed me something they had done, I would expect *them* to report on how well they had done it, and would write down what they said, and invite them to sign it. At first they offered back the kind of praise they might have anticipated from me: 'It's really beautiful and you really like it Mrs Brooker!' but quite quickly they became more self-critical, of their own and then each other's work. Because they sometimes had to wait to talk to me, they often turned to each other for comment, and I heard both generous praise and thoughtful criticisms being offered:

That's really nice, your mum's gonna like your writing!
I wish I could do a Batman like that ...

Is that number 5 the right way round?

Some children found the new regime harder than others: Roisin, whose older sister had explained the rules of school to her particularly thoroughly, cried because she couldn't have a star (there had never been any stars) and took to drawing her own stars on anything she drew or wrote. But the transformation was surprisingly easy, once I had learned to control my own thoughtless habits. By the end of the year the children were realistic and confident both in appraising their own efforts, and in communicating their views to others. To my subjective and unscientific eye, they seemed more independent, motivated and mutually supportive than any class I had taught. Whether or not this was the case, the events of that year made a permanent impression on me.

Assessment: *the* what *and* why, where *and* when, who *and* how

Transitions are key moments for assessing children. We expect, and hope, that every time a child moves into a new setting, some form of information is passed on from the previous setting. We assume too that the child's new care giver or teacher will make her own formal or informal assessments of the child. We may be less conscious however of the impact of 'being assessed' on a child's well-being and development.

Most early years practitioners, of course, make such assessments all the time they are with children. From their first day in a Babies' room, children are subject to our observations of their development and learning, their personalities and preferences. This may be the only period in which young children are unaware of the assessments professionals make of them; once they are 2 or 3, children know that we are writing notes on what they do, and may begin to share in the record which documents their interests and achievements. From their entry into formal schooling, as the last chapter showed, many children are only too aware of the hierarchies of achievements and approval that count in their settings. Learning about your own place in that hierarchy may be one of the hardest lessons of successive transitions.

What and why?

The *what* of early record keeping is holistic and inclusive, from feeding and toileting to sleeping and smiling. It is a record of well-being that ideally contributes to well-being. As children move on, they are increasingly subject to normative expectations about the ages at which certain stages of development will appear. In England the *Birth to Three Matters* Framework (DfES 2002) introduced a structure for observing children's development as a strong, independent, active learner and communicator, while the *Curriculum Guidance* (DfES/QCA 2001) for the 3–5 age phase included 'stepping stones' towards goals to be achieved at the age of 5 or 6. At the point of transition from the Reception class to Year 1 of formal schooling, children's numerical scores on the *Foundation Stage Profile* (DfES 2003) were recorded for the first – but not the last – time in their school career. And from Year 1, the National Curriculum expectations for each child in each subject area became the dominant mode of assessment, so that 'working towards Level One' became an indicator of low achievement, rather than a simple descriptor of a child's current levels of understanding.

Because it is demanding for practitioners, this increasingly formal and complex system of assessment requirements has an impact on the experiences of children. As time goes by they may be set 'tasks' designed to produce evidence of their knowledge, skills and understanding. Before we know it, or intend it, children become aware that there is a right and a wrong answer to the questions adults put to them, and that they themselves are acquiring the identity, in their school or setting, of someone who generally gets things right, or does not.

The *why* of assessment has increasingly crept up and ambushed early years' practitioners, who have traditionally viewed assessment as 'for the child', or parents, but may now be obliged by regulations to view it as 'for the school or setting', or for the governing body or committee, or for the inspector. At heart, early years' educators believe in assessing young children's development and learning as a means of planning appropriate provision for the child, or considering helpful interventions. But as early education becomes 'schoolified' (Bennett 2006), children's assessments may be seen as a form of accountability, a means of demonstrating that the teacher and the school are doing their job properly. Drummond (2003) has argued that no single assessment can serve a range of different and possibly conflicting purposes; that an assessment carried out 'for the child' – to identify interests and schemas, or to plan 'next steps' – will not be adequate for the inspectors. Adults working with young children have to hold on tight to their principles when they are confronted by such demands.

Where and when?

The narrowing of focus which tends to happen as children go through the system – from a holistic and inclusive perspective to a numerical one

– is accompanied by a narrowing of the times and places where assessment occurs. In infancy and early childhood, children may be observed at any moment of the day, and in any place where they find themselves: it would be interesting to know what proportion of child observations is undertaken in the gardens and outdoor areas, and the snack rooms and sleep rooms, of settings for young children. This is because what is observed and recorded is *whatever the child does* or *whatever interests the child*. With older pre-school children, the cumulative evidence gathered in portfolios – discussed later – takes this principle even further, as children not only select their activities, but select which of them they wish to have documented.

The breadth and depth of such observations is typically lost as children's assessments become regulated by profiles or checklists, goals or stepping stones, informing us of *what the child knows* or *what the child can do (unaided)*. The introduction of a formal academic curriculum, usually in the first year of the primary or elementary school, may be accompanied by the introduction of formal tests such as the Standard Assessment Tasks of the English National Curriculum, which children 'sit' on a particular day in a specially ordered classroom that enables them to write their answers in silence and without 'copying'. The impact of such explicit testing on children's confidence and their identity, as they make the transition into grades where tests are held, concerns many teachers.

The notion of 'school readiness', as we have seen, permeates school systems around the world (Arnold et al. 2006) and has been particularly contested in the USA, where the idea of 'children being ready for school' is challenged by an emphasis on 'schools being ready for children'. Where 'readiness checklists' operate, as Kagan (1999: 2) reports,

> Parents worry over whether their children will be *ready* for school; teachers wrestle with whether they will be greeted by a *ready* group of children; and policymakers wonder if they have produced the policies and programs that will magically make children *ready* for school.

Presumably all this anxiety does not pass over the heads of the children themselves.

Who and how?

A parallel reduction in the range of those eligible to assess the child accompanies these developments. Small children may be observed and described with confidence by everyone who knows them – parents, grandparents and siblings, neighbours and friends, and key workers: everyone is an expert, because everything about the child is interesting. Many pre-school settings work hard to sustain this inclusive stance, involving children and their peers, as well as family members and co-workers, in constructing the record. But as the content of the evaluation becomes more formal and more academic in focus, the necessary expertise seemingly becomes concentrated in the hands of professional educators. Parents of 5-year-olds, as well as the children themselves, may fear to show their ignorance of the relationship between graphemes and phonemes, and children are unlikely to regard themselves as experts, or as competent judges of their own learning.

In England, the move from the Early Years Foundation Stage (2007) to Year 1 begins a slow shift from broadly documented early learning to the narrowly defined 'Learning Outcomes' which will lead, in Year 2, to the 'tests'. Despite children's appetite for change, challenge and 'hard work', it is difficult to see how they can maintain a sense of control over their own learning within this framework. For this to be achieved we need to take several steps backward, and look more closely at the theory and practice of early assessments.

Understanding assessment

The sociologist Basil Bernstein, as well as developing some very complex formal frameworks for analysing school processes, offered some very simple insights into the underlying sources of these processes. Schools, he explained, are a 'message system' made up of three components – curriculum, pedagogy, and evaluation – all of which are equally powerful in their impact on children's development and learning (Bernstein 1975). When considering transitions we are very alert to the 'messages' conveyed by the curriculum and the pedagogy of schools and settings, but may be less aware of the impact of evaluation methods.

Children's expectations and evaluations

Research has demonstrated a number of ways that evaluation has an effect on children's identity, and their dispositions to be life-long learners. One of the most important areas of study has been into the foundations of children's own 'learning dispositions', the attitudes they hold about themselves as learners, and their beliefs about the purposes of learning. A series of studies in the 1980s and 1990s (Dweck and Leggett 1988; Ames 1992) identified two different 'types' of children, based on their engagement with learning and especially their response to difficulties, and tracked these typical beliefs and behaviours back to children's beliefs about the importance of intelligence and effort:

- Children with a 'mastery' orientation were interested in acquiring knowledge and skills for their own sake: they wished to learn more, to *improve* on their current abilities, for the satisfaction of doing so, rather than for the satisfaction of pleasing others and receiving praise.
- Children with a 'helpless' orientation were less interested in knowledge and skills for their own sake, and were more keen to *prove* their abilities to others such as teachers and peers; they attempted tasks with the aim of receiving praise and commendation from others

'Mastery' children are described as holding 'learning goals'. They enjoy learning in the school or pre-school setting because they tackle new challenges without anxiety, learn from their own mistakes, and are keen to attempt again something that has gone wrong the first time. Their positive attitude is associated with a belief that success comes through effort: if you get something wrong it is not because you are inadequate but because you need to try again or try harder. They value the *process* rather than the product.

Here is Kelly, demonstrating her mastery disposition while undertaking a 'baseline assessment' task at All Saints':

Kelly, along with her classmates, was being assessed on a baseline measure of completing simple jigsaw puzzles. She was experienced with puzzles after spending a year in nursery, and progressed rapidly through the array of increasingly difficult puzzles the staff had set out, seizing a new puzzle with one hand as she fitted the last piece to the previous one and pushed it away from her. Having exhausted them she quickly improvised her own challenge, turning a 12-piece puzzle upside down (so that the picture was hidden) and announcing 'Now I'm going to do it the hard way'. She completed the puzzle by trial and error, with considerable effort and concentration, and instructed the researcher, 'Now you mix some of them up for me while I shut my eyes, to make it harder this time'. Eventually she tried putting some puzzles together, by feel, with her eyes still closed; after several failed attempts, when she remarked 'I've done it wrong, I'll have to have another go', she gave up and pranced away without further concern. At no time did she seem interested in the adult's view of her performance.

(Brooker and Broadbent 2007: 55)

'Helpless' children are described as holding 'performance goals'. Their classroom learning is less enjoyable and successful because they try to avoid difficult or challenging situations, and make excuses to cover up for their own mistakes. Their negative attitude is associated with a belief that success is a result of innate and unchangeable aspects of their own identity: if you get something wrong it is a sign that you are stupid or inadequate, and trying again is probably pointless. They focus on the *product* of an activity rather than the process.

Some of Kelly's classmates resorted to a range of ingenious excuses when offered a jigsaw they did not wish to attempt, and a few showed real discomfort and resistance. As an observer of the following entry assessment (recorded by her class teacher), I was convinced that Tuhura's lack of cooperation masked a lack of familiarity and confidence:

Task: tray puzzles

Tuhura needed 'persuading' to attempt jigsaws; very unco-operative; needs more practice and teaching; not fully concentrated and looks around the room when trying to fit pieces into spaces.

As Smiley and Dweck (1994) have shown, in situations like this 'helpless' children typically opt for the easiest puzzle or offer to do one they have already successfully completed, while 'mastery' children seek to try their skills on more difficult problems.

Children's beliefs about the reasons for their success or failure – their attributions to innate intelligence, or continuing effort – tend to reflect the beliefs of their family and community, but are further shaped by their school experiences: it has been shown that 'helpless' children can acquire a mastery orientation in the right supportive environment. But the combined experience of transition into a new setting, and being 'tested' on their knowledge and skills by a new adult, may reinforce a tendency to pursue performance goals rather than learning goals. Classrooms which value competitive rather than collaborative efforts foster this tendency to 'negative affect directed toward the self' (Ames 1992, cited in Gipps 2002: 81). An additional problem however may be an undue focus on the *individual*, and this is discussed later.

Teacher expectations

We have known for a long time about the immediate and long-term effects of 'teacher expectation' – those subtle but insidious evaluations of a child or group which may mean that they are viewed as less capable, offered less access to learning, and challenged less than 'more capable' children. The early classic studies (Rosenthal and Jacobson 1968; Rist 1970) offered glaring examples of the consequences for children of early misjudgements. In Rosenthal and Jacobson's case, this was because the teacher was deliberately misinformed by the researchers, but in Rist's case the misjudgement was the outcome of a teacher's own prejudices and assumptions. The teacher in the class of 'ghetto children' he observed placed children into ability groups based on their appearance (including the darkness of their skin), their address, their parent's employment and affluence, the correctness of their spoken English, and the family's reputation in the school. These allocations were made in the first few days of kindergarten, and persisted through the first three years that the children attended school. Rist concluded that the teacher had an 'ideal type' of the successful pupil in her head, and sorted the children in her class, unintentionally, according to their closeness to this type.

Such extreme cases may be unusual, but English studies suggest that 'teacher expectation effects' are hard to eliminate. Barbara Tizard's (1988) study of infant schools showed that the gap between different groups of children widened as they went through school, as a result of teachers' judgements, while Waterhouse's (1991) study of informal assessments at the start of Reception shows that pupil identities are formed during their first few days of school, based on the teacher's idea of how a 'normal' pupil behaves. We might argue that such imprecise and often inaccurate judgements are precisely why we need to have detailed assessments of children but we would then have to ask, who makes these assessments, and on what basis? Unless we believe in the possibility of a wholly fair, objective and constructive evaluation of children, there is no escape from the bias which has informed many children's early categorizations, and we have to look for alternative approaches and solutions. Once again, it must be assumed that children are aware of their teacher's view of them, and the evidence is that many children bring their performance into line with this view.

The effects of praise

Early years practitioners are conscious of the impact of self-esteem on children's development and learning, and are often at pains to build self-esteem through praise (Roberts 2002). They argue that 'you can't give enough praise' and that 'feeling good about themselves' is the key to children's learning. All teachers know too that in the short term at least, praise is an infallible mechanism for individual motivation and whole-class behaviour management (Hitz and Driscoll 1988). But reliance on this mechanism means ignoring some unpalatable truths:

- Teachers' legitimacy to confer praise on children implies that they are the sole arbiters of children's behaviour, knowledge, skills, learning, and effort: if an adult praises your painting there is no need for you to evaluate it yourself.
- This legitimacy is automatically accompanied by the right to criticize or make negative comments on the child's effort, behaviour and so on: again, if this right resides with adults a child need not bother to develop the necessary skills and strategies to self-evaluate.
- Teachers' praise takes control of their learning away from children, who have no voice in the matter but simply do as they are told: they become increasingly dependent, rather than increasingly independent, as learners.
- Public praise – the kind most frequently offered in classrooms – prompts the kinds of social comparisons between children which damage both their self-esteem and their learning dispositions.

As the Valley School study showed, some children are already 'praise junkies' when they start formal schooling; they make comparisons and compete on an individual basis, and need to be weaned off a rewards system which reinforces their 'helpless' disposition, their need to *prove* themselves to peers and teachers.

Children's own expectations of the 'rules of school' include the notions of success and failure, winners and losers, and some schools and classrooms build on these expectations – they make some (but not all) children biddable and docile. But with every subsequent transition children experience fewer opportunities for intrinsic motivation, and more opportunities for extrinsic rewards. If we wish to hand children control over their own learning, as well as their behaviour, we need to investigate other ways to assess.

Children in control of their learning

Many recent initiatives in curriculum and pedagogy are founded in the belief that children should retain control of their own learning as they move through the early years of schooling. This raises the question of whether it is possible to devise assessment practices which similarly leave control of the learning agenda in the child's hands. As Carr et al. (2005: 140) explain:

Traditionally, the balance of power between teacher and child or pupil during assessment has been very one-sided. The teacher writes the assessment, makes an interpretation, perhaps discusses it with other teachers and the family, but the child is not part of the equation.

Their response has been to redefine the purposes as well as the methods of assessment: to make it many sided, or multi-voiced.

Principles for pre-school assessment

Researchers and theorists working to unpick and redress the imbalance of power created by traditional assessments point to a number of key principles which may serve to transform the 'messages' conveyed to children during assessment:

1. Traditional assessments are designed to measure what a child can do unaided and unsupported; child-friendly assessments look for what a child is capable of *with the support of others* (Gipps 2002). In this way, they can be seen as 'assessment for tomorrow' (Fleer and Richardson 2004: 121) rather than assessment of the past. What 'tomorrow' holds describes the child's capability in the Zone of Proximal Development (ZPD), which is more important for learning than the child's current or 'actual' development.
2. Traditional assessments measure the child's learning *as an individual*, free of social and cultural context; sociocultural assessments recognize that learning takes place socially, in a cultural and historical context, and is shared among a group of learners. Hence it is argued that assessment like learning should be 'distributed' across the social group, with children assisting each other in reaching conclusions (Carr et al. 2005).
3. Traditional assessment measures what matters and is relevant to the teacher; child-friendly assessment should attend to what matters and is relevant to the child. Claxton (1995: 340) argues that it must include all the situations in which 'learners are developing their sense of what counts as "good work" for themselves – where it is some inner sense of satisfaction, which is the touchstone of quality ... rather than the application of rules'. Only by valuing what the child values can assessment give the children control of their own learning.
4. Traditional assessments isolate the individual child, and produce competition and comparison between children; child-friendly assessments produce collaboration and solidarity between children. In the words of Cowie and Carr (2004: 96) they should help to

'conscript' children into a community of learners with a shared purpose and culture which promotes a sense of competence and continuity (the goals of transitions)

5. Traditional assessments are undertaken by one 'expert'; child-friendly assessments are shared between the teacher, family and friends of the child, and always involve the contribution of children themselves

6. Traditional assessments measure discrete items of knowledge and skills – cutting with scissors, completing a puzzle, naming letters; child-friendly assessments describe the child's *dispositions towards learning*, and their *participation* in the setting.

Rogoff argues that what should be assessed is children's 'process of participation in community activities' (1998, cited in Fleer 2004: 112), as they move from being 'peripheral' members of their learning community to being full members. In this view, children's growing involvement in activities, their growing sense of belonging to the group, and their growing contributions to the group culture, are the significant signs of learning. The difficult question, though, is whether the innovative assessment practices developed in pre-schools can, or even should, be continued through the transition into formal schooling.

Pre-school practice: (i) High/Scope

High/Scope methods and principles have travelled the world since they were first devised, in Michigan in the 1970s, as one of the 'planned variations' of Project Head Start. The success of the movement is reinforced by an unparalleled long-term research record – the earliest High/Scope participants are now in their 40s, but the evidence of the benefits they retain from their early experiences can still be identified (Schweinhart et al. 2004). The programme has a complex array of cognitive targets, and is founded on some quite formal and individualistic beliefs about the ways children learn, which not all early educators would now agree with. But some of its fundamental principles have turned out to be so important – and so simple – that they have been incorporated into other curricula and other programmes in the intervening decades. The most important of these is the well-known 'Plan–Do–Review' sequence; a less familiar principle is that no child is praised, at least publicly, for their efforts or successes.

The High/Scope Plan–Do–Review sequence, which was revolutionary in the 1970s, now seems disarmingly simple. In every session the children first engage in a planning meeting or activity, where their intentions for the session are recorded; they then have a work-time in which to carry out the chosen activity (or not), and the session ends with a review meeting in which children describe what was attempted, and what was achieved – 'how it went' – to an adult or peers. Behind this simple sequence is David Weikart's powerful notion that for a child of 3 or 4 to plan ahead – sometimes even to plan for tomorrow – and to be held responsible for those plans and their execution, represents a huge cognitive challenge which most children respond to extremely well. In the 'review', guided by well-trained practitioners, children can discuss, not only their successes or failures, but the suitability of their plans, and the resources they needed to carry them out. The sequence can be viewed as a recipe for inculcating realistic and positive learning dispositions; for establishing a locus of control within the child; and for freeing the child from an undue reliance on adult judgements. This latter priority has been incorporated into the High/Scope training, which inducts practitioners into the practice of withholding praise and public evaluation: children are helped to self-evaluate, and their objectives and successes may be discussed with them, but the final verdict on their success or failure is the child's own.

As the research has demonstrated, the impact of such a programme on learning dispositions in early childhood has life-long consequences: in their 40s, the earliest High/Scope 'graduates' continue to outstrip control groups in their education and employment records, their avoidance of criminal convictions, and their positive attitudes to society. But this is no magic bullet: it is simply one example of the application of child-friendly principles to early childhood programmes; and other examples are equally well known.

(ii) Reggio Emilia: documentation

The pre-primary schools of Reggio Emilia in northern Italy have enjoyed a similarly world-wide reputation, and similar attempts at replication, since they first came to the attention of practitioners and researchers in other countries in the 1980s. For many of those who admire the Reggio practice, but can see the problems with transposing a North Italian culture into other international contexts, the defining practice which *can* be transposed, or at least adapted, to other settings is the ongoing assessment practice known as *documentation*.

Documentation is a continuous record of children's thinking and activity as they engage in group projects, described in essence as 'making learning visible' (Rinaldi 2005). Rather than assessing the child's knowledge, skills and understandings against the requirements of a pre-set curriculum or statutory objectives, the educators engage in continuous dialogue with children about the development of their ideas and interests: the ongoing work on a project or activity is recorded as it happens, through children's drawings and photographs and the record of their discussions and, most importantly, in an iterative process, these 'documents' are regularly reviewed with the group of children, so that the progress of their thinking and making is continually updated. The resulting record becomes a document for everyone to view: it is shared with parents and other educators (and also, though this may be less helpful, with the hordes of international visitors who tour the schools each year).

However distant the Reggio approach may seem to be from the mainstream pre-school and school practices of other regions, the principles on which documentation is based are wholly matched to the 'child-friendly' understanding of assessment which this chapter advocates. This mode of assessment:

- Begins with children's own ideas, interests and motivations, and serves the children's interests (in every sense) before considering those of the adults, the curriculum or the school.
- Values all the different 'languages' that children use to communicate – modelling, exploring and dancing, as well as speaking and writing and recording.
- Supports and values group learning and the shared development of ideas: what is documented is not a single child's progress towards understanding, but a process of shared thinking within a small community of learners.
- Locates evaluation within the child or children: adults do not 'pass judgement' on children's thinking, they simply attend, inquire and document the ideas and achievements of the children themselves.
- Provides a springboard towards the 'next steps' in children's development, by helping them to know what they know (metacognition) and identify those things they do not yet know, but may wish to know.

The precise form that documentation takes in the Reggio pre-schools may not and need not be replicated in other settings, but the principles on which it is based resonate with recent understandings of assessment in other locations. In the view of the educators, the children's experience of controlling their own learning gives them an 'extra pocket' (of resources and resilience) to dip into when they move into conventional primary schools.

(iii) Te Whaariki: learning stories

The New Zealand early childhood curriculum, *Te Whaariki* (New Zealand Ministry of Education 1996), which was discussed in Chapter 4, sets new challenges for assessment: like High/Scope, the programme has detailed cognitive and curriculum goals for children but places more emphasis on the broader dispositions that they display. These dispositions – belonging, well-being, exploring, communicating and contributing – are assessed by means of 'learning stories', observation-based narratives which are typically constructed by the adults in the setting, shared with the child and parents, and used as the basis for 'what next?' decisions. The aim, in Carr's (2001) words, is to help children to be *ready, willing and able* to learn. By this she means that the child is in possession of the necessary knowledge and skills, and the necessary human and material resources, for learning, but also of a sense of confidence in the rightness of this environment and this moment as a time and place to act.

Learning stories can be written about children from infancy through to school age, and like the documentation employed in Reggio and elsewhere, they can be shared and extended by the involvement of the child, parents and other community members. The child's learning is not *private* – something that happens inside the child's head, and can be tested by tasks and questions – but belongs to everyone in the learning community: family and friends, members of the *whanau* or supportive network, make their own contributions to the record of the child's growing competence as a learner and communicator. The ownership of the record also lies with the children and their families, who take the portfolio with them as the child moves into the next stage of the education system.

As with all other forms of good pre-school practice, holistic assessment should serve at least two purposes: it should support the child's learning *in the present* – by empowering the child and family, linking home and setting, and enabling appropriate planning to take place; and it should support children's transition into a new setting, by helping them to acquire the resources they will need for successive stages in their educational journey. The 'readiness' which Carr advocates cannot be measured by a checklist of letter-names and number-bonds, but through a shared understanding of the goals of education.

(iv) Good practice in pre-school

Personal portfolios
In recent years, pre-school settings everywhere have increasingly adapted the child-friendly ideas of innovative international programmes to suit their own settings and their own practice. In the UK, most maintained settings document the individual child's learning through portfolios of photographs, drawings and written commentary in which children's interests, involvement, persistence and collaboration are recorded and discussed, and their 'next steps' are planned. Children and parents are invited to contribute to the individual record, and the family is encouraged to bring the portfolio with them into their next classroom (where it may not always be welcomed by the teacher, who has her own busy agenda for her new class).

Video links
Innovative centres such as the Pen Green Centre (Whalley 2007) also use video as the medium for regular exchanges and dialogue between the child, the family and the centre. Videos made at nursery are discussed with parents, who are encouraged to identify their children's schemas and track them in their observation of the child's interests at home; the recordings made by parents are subsequently brought back into the setting and form part of staff planning for the children, thus completing the 'Pen Green Loop' of shared evaluation. All these methods support the learning of individual children and provide each of them with multiple close links between their home and pre-school settings, enhancing their sense of well-being and belonging, and their opportunities to develop competence.

Group work
Many pre-schools also celebrate the learning of small groups through joint activities, and jointly constructed displays of investigations and outcomes, in which individual children's ideas and problem solving have contributed to a shared learning experience: *How we found out what the snails like to eat; What happened when we made a house for Joel's Batman; We wanted to know how big our feet are.* In environments where collaborative learning like this is valued, the assessment of joint achievements genuinely values the participation of every member of the group. Some children are good at ideas, some at organizing, some at cutting, some at sticking, some at locating resources, some at asking for adult help: joint activity reinforces the idea that all children's participation is valued even if every child's contribution is unique. Those individual contributions

may of course be recorded on children's individual checklists or profiles (if that is what the system requires), but the children's *experience* of being assessed, assessing themselves and assessing each other, is a positive contribution to their learning and to their formation of an identity as a learner – an identity which is often challenged during transitions.

Assessment in school classrooms

Transitions into new phases of education should reflect the transformation of children's abilities as they grow. Just as learning environments need to change their own 'readiness' as children engage in new modes of thinking, so do the ways that learning is assessed: the acquisition of certain kinds of 'subject knowledge' through the school years can only be properly supported by teachers who can identify what pupils have achieved, individually, and where they need additional resources, as individuals. In spite of innovative projects to assess older pupils' knowledge and skills through group projects and problem solving, it is almost inevitable that society will continue to require individual test scores and exam results as it channels children into different levels and 'streams' of our complex and competitive education systems. So it is right that the assessment of school-age learning should be different from that of pre-school learning. But how different?

A whole research industry has been built on developing assessment instruments, or tests, which aim to be fair, accurate, culturally neutral and even enjoyable for school pupils (Tymms and Merrell 2004), and more recently, the principle of 'assessment for learning', rather than assessment *of* learning, has shaped research and practice (Black et al. 2004). There is no space here to discuss the debates that have resulted. Instead I want to consider, briefly, the extent to which assessment in more formal classrooms might be informed by the principles developed by pre-school educators. Assessment practices in schools should embody similar respect for children's identities as learners; similar attention to children's future learning rather than their current level; similar involvement of children as assessors; and similar recognition of children's participation in group as well as individual activities. Like pre-school classrooms, school classes should enable children to be 'conscripted' as Cowie and Carr (2004) describe it, into a community of learners where they can view themselves as people who investigate, communicate and contribute to the achievement of the whole group.

Children's identity as learners

> Because of the public nature of much questioning and feedback in
> the classroom, and the power dynamic in the teacher-student
> relationship, assessment plays a key role in identity formation. The
> language of assessment and evaluation is one of the routes by which
> the identity of young persons is formed.
>
> (Gipps 2002: 80)

Examining the nature of formative and summative assessment in primary schools raises several issues about the impact of current practice on
children's view of themselves as learners, and the ways that this practice
may need to change if transitions are not to weaken children's dispositions to learn.

Feedback and motivation

As research has shown, many of the differentials that grow up between
children, or between groups, in school classrooms, are attributable to the
form of teacher feedback that they receive. Tunstall and Gipps (1996)
constructed a typology of the kinds of positive and negative feedback
that were given to children aged 6 and 7, and the same typology was
applied by Burrell and Bubb (2000) to children aged 4 and 5. The latter
study demonstrated clearly that children who had adapted well in the
transition to school received high levels of positive ('rewarding' and
'approving') feedback from their teachers, while children described by
teachers as 'poorly adjusted' received mainly negative ('disapproving' or
even 'punishing') feedback on their efforts. One 'poorly adjusted' girl
received 13 disapproving comments on her work during a single day,
and overall 'more negative feedback was recorded than positive feedback' (Burrell and Bubb 2000: 62). It is hard to imagine a similar scenario
in a pre-school setting.

Black and Wiliam (1998: 9) explain the links between negative feedback of this kind, and children's self-belief as learners: 'Pupils who
encounter difficulties and poor results are led to believe that they lack
ability, and this belief leads them to attribute their difficulties to a defect
in themselves about which they cannot do a great deal'. As in Dweck's
earlier studies (Dweck and Leggett 1988), the experiences of difficulty or
failure which dishearten children in the short term may strengthen
negative dispositions in the longer term, as children come to view
themselves as unsuccessful learners.

Evaluating a narrowly defined curriculum

> One of the greatest challenges facing educationalists in using a sociocultural perspective for assessment is the current testing regime advocated in many English-speaking countries around the world.
>
> (Fleer 2002: 114)

Marilyn Fleer's argument for sociocultural assessment incorporates all the notions of learning as social and collaborative, shared and situated, that we met in relation to pre-school environments, and clearly this perspective on learning is hard to reconcile with a view of assessment as 'tests'. It is in the nature of tests to measure narrowly defined outcomes and to require responses which are either right or wrong. By contrast, in most pre-school settings, children's individual, provisional, amateur, hypothetical conclusions are valued and taken seriously, and children's questions are as important as their answers. Fleer (2002: 115) continues:

> Documenting individual test scores, then compiling test scores into sets of results for classrooms, schools and finally an entire system does little to inform *how* teaching practices must change for the improvement of outcomes ... As most educators are aware, it is simplistic to think that by assessing individuals somehow improvements in outcomes for children will result ...

The tests – formal or informal – that many school children are set, could be regarded as useless but trivial, since they tell teachers so little about children's real capabilities. But they are more than trivial if they have an impact on children's own view of themselves as successful learners, or on teachers' beliefs about the child's potential. In the All Saints' study (Brooker 2002), assessments designed to be child friendly, and conducted by kindly and sympathetic individuals, probably had little immediate effect on the children themselves, but did contribute to a construction of some children as deficient in the basic knowledge, skills and attitudes required to be a pupil, and had a subsequent impact on the way the curriculum was offered to these children, as this example of a 'baseline assessment task' shows:

Task (maths): Sorts objects using one criterion

Jemma was invited to 'sort' some jumbled farm-animals into 'fields'; she chose to assemble in one field a cat, a farmer, a chicken and some sheep. The conversation then went:

Liz: *Is that how you want them to go ...? Great ... why did you choose those ones for that field?*
Jemma: *Because they friends.*
Liz: *Oh, right, good, are they?*

When my notes on this event were transferred to the assessment report, Jemma was officially recorded as 'unable to sort'.

From this point on, and on the basis of a narrow definition of the meaning of 'sorting' like and unlike objects, Jemma was presumed to have limited understanding of mathematics.

Understanding school tasks

What Jemma really lacked was an understanding of what 'school' and teachers actually required of her – what Bourdieu (1986) calls 'cultural capital'. Cultural capital consists not simply of the subject-knowledge and study-skills that are valued in classrooms, but of the knowledge *about* school which children acquire through their early experiences and in the context of their home *habitus* (see Chapter 3). Jemma did not realize that when a teacher or researcher asks you to sort animals into fields, she really means 'show me that you can put all the same ones together'; naturally she knew very well how to 'sort' the things that mattered to her, in the real world. Sorting farm animals, which may seem like a child-friendly and interesting task, is both unfamiliar and artificial to children who have never played with toy animals, or never been on a farm. Jemma's Bangladeshi classmates were even more confused by this task, but like her they all knew how to sort the objects in their own environment.

Research into assessment in primary classrooms shows again and again how children misunderstand and misinterpret teachers' intentions and their cues and 'clues': Torrance and Pryor (2004) offer a moment-by-moment analysis of an episode in which a teacher offers 'helpful' hints to enable her reception class to arrive at the right answers about the story of the Three Bears. These same children may have recently left an environment in which their own ideas were welcomed and valued, rather than judged against the answers in the teacher's mind. One of the most important tasks for them as they go through school will be to learn what teachers expect of them.

What 'learning' do we value?

So long as schools hold different values from pre-schools, their assessment methods will be equally different. There is a revolution in our conception of school knowledge (Wells and Claxton 2002) but it is a long time coming: as Wells and Claxton argue, learning in the 21st century needs to be about change and uncertainty rather than about fixed understandings. The skills and dispositions children will need in this century will be the ability to think in a lateral rather than linear mode; to accept uncertainty and entertain conflicting perspectives; to work collaboratively rather than competitively; to think along divergent paths, rather than follow the paths trodden by others.

To this extent, Jemma's answer could be seen as a good one. But in many of our classrooms, children like her may continue to find that they are the kinds of children who get the wrong answer; and teachers may continue to act on similar assumptions. A rethinking, not of specific practices for assessment but of common principles for assessment across different phases, might allow children and schools to be more ready for each other.

7

Transitions for life

How do you learn things?
Messages go through your brain and tell you things: when you read
you look at the books and read what the letters say because you've got
a mouth on your brain and a long hose pipe goes to your ear ... the
hands in your brain get the messages in your brain and roll them up,
and the water pipes carry them all the way down to your face.
I leave my brain in a cup at night because you have to don't think
things at night do you?.

(Andrew, 4 years 10 months)

We think about the words it says in the books, in your head: my brain
keeps it in somewhere safe – I keep words and books and sometimes I
keep paintings in my brain.

(Abiola, 5 years)

In drawing together the many threads that run through this book, and
trying to weave from them a recipe for 'good practice' in supporting
young children's transitions, I am conscious of the need to return continually to where I started: to understanding the nature of transitions,
and the goals of transitions, in order to develop good insights into the
kinds of support that children and families require. I will begin by
referring to one more important metaphor that has been used to define
transitions – the idea of 'transplanting' from one place to another – but
will go on to argue that a rather different model seems more appropriate
for the 21st-century world. In working through this model I will consider

what can be done, by policy-makers, providers, practitioners and parents, to ensure that early transitions really are positive steps towards life-long learning and well-being for children. The book ends on a positive note, because the evidence is that children's well-being is gaining greater priority in many societies, and that transitions are now an issue of global interest.

Transitions and transplanting

Chapter 3 introduced the idea that the environments in which children live their early years should be understood as cultures, in the sense of 'environments designed to produce optimal growth and development in the young'. An extension of this idea is to consider transitions – from one culture to another – as a form of transplanting, similar to the transplanting of young plants and seedlings. Cleave et al. (1982) were the first to compare the process to the task of a gardener moving seedlings from smaller to larger growing environments: they pointed out that young plants need more space and more stimulus if they are to grow and flourish, but that transplanting needs to be undertaken skilfully and expertly so that the shock does not set the plant back (or worse). Julie Fisher (2006) has skilfully developed this theme, describing in detail both the careful preparation that is needed before transplanting – including an awareness of the strengths and weaknesses of individuals (children or plants) – and the careful nurture that is required before, during and after the process. In both instances the 'responsible adults' are expected to use their expertise to prepare the environments and make the best possible arrangements. The desired outcomes in both instances, of course, are strong, healthy and increasingly independent organisms.

Two approaches to supporting transitions

The image of the careful gardener, though appealing and appropriate, does not quite capture for me the reality of children's lives in modern societies. As earlier chapters have discussed, children are often required to make continual frequent transitions from one environment to another, and these environments themselves may also be in a state of continuous flux and change. Fthenakis (1998) reminds us that changes in the lives of individuals – ontogenetic changes – take place within the context of changes in the life of human societies – phylogenetic changes – so that any adequate model of change needs to be a dynamic one. The adults, both parents and practitioners, who are engaged in supporting children's transitions may themselves feel they are simultaneously 'running to catch up' with changes in their own personal and professional lives.

So I am abandoning the metaphor of the gardener, and considering instead two other similar but distinct approaches to supporting transitions. The first is the 'readiness' model, while the second might be called a 'positive outcomes' model.

Supporting transitions: the 'readiness' model

> The relative importance of school readiness and ready schools is much debated.
>
> (Bennett 2006: 11)

This first approach has been referred to throughout the book and needs little further explanation. Its two strands or strategies – 'ready children' and 'ready schools' – have developed alongside each other in the last few years, very explicitly in the USA and more implicitly elsewhere (Arnold et al. 2006; Bennett 2006). The former strand, which placed responsibility for a successful transition on the individual child and family, assumed that children should prepare for school by somehow acquiring a complete toolkit of accomplishments, a set of physical, social and cognitive skills which would enable them to 'start school ready to learn' (National Education Goals Panel 1991). Children who did not meet the assessment criteria were sometimes refused entry to school and admitted a year later than their peer group. As Kagan (1999: 2) reported, 'in the United States readiness for school is a high-stakes event', and she argued that the discussion of what children really need to know at the start of school should be undertaken by parents and practitioners rather than policy makers. Meanwhile, the mere concept that any child might *not* be 'ready to learn' – from birth, rather than from the age of 5 – is one which parents and early educators, as well as developmental psychologists, will reject out of hand.

At the end of the 1990s, a survey of representatives in all 50 American states (Saluja et al. 2000) showed that most had been persuaded of the unfairness of this practice, and that six explicitly placed their emphasis on 'schools being ready for all children'. But these authors report two outstanding concerns: that at the local (rather than state-wide) level, the continued use and abuse of standardized 'readiness' assessments' might be harmful for children, and that 'the second side of the equation – the readiness of schools – is not being widely assessed' (2000: 12).

We have encountered many ways that schools and settings can be ready for children. They include *knowing* children as individuals through careful inquiries and observation, *listening* to children as they become involved in activities, *making relationships* with parents, and *respecting* the goals and values of local communities. But despite these defining criteria, the rhetoric still seems a long way from the reality. Unless policy makers and legislators, at the national or local level, can require providers to implement the necessary changes in school culture, the blame for some children's poor start in school may continue to be placed on the child and family.

Although the model of schools ready for children, and children ready for schools, seems an attractive one, it can also seem both negative (in its view of transitions) and limited (in its focus on cognition). 'Readiness' offers a solution to a 'problem'; a means to manage a one-off transition; an overall goal of adjustment, adaptation and 'getting it over with'. Though designed to ease children's transition into learning, it fundamentally suggests that the process of transition is an obstacle to learning, rather than an opportunity. For this reason I propose a slightly different, and more positive, alternative.

Supporting transitions: the 'positive outcomes' model

Taking a positive, rather than negative, view of transitions requires a shift in perspective from ideas of 'readiness', though it depends similarly on a two-pronged focus for action: working with schools and settings, and working with children. This approach takes the view *not* that transitions are a problem to be managed, but that transitions are an important opportunity for learning; *not* that the transition is a one-off event, but that growing and learning through transitions is a vital and permanent feature of human lives. The two strategies implied by this model are: (i) mediating the discontinuities between phases (working with schools and settings) and (ii) supporting the development of resources for change (working with children). The goals of this approach might be those summarized by Ramey and Ramey (1998: 295): 'a lifetime love of learning ... a society of competent, cooperative and contributing citizens'. In other words: children who perceive themselves as strong and successful learners, and who work together to solve problems and manage their environments in a changing world.

Strategies for 'positive outcomes': (i) mediating discontinuities

The problems of discontinuities between phases and locations, and some of the current solutions, were discussed in Chapter 4. It is important to emphasize that this approach is not about erasing the differences between settings, which are key to children's continuing development, but about mediating the unnecessarily abrupt discontinuities that frequently result from the *ad hoc* and unplanned development of our education systems. This task requires action at many levels, from policy makers to practitioners: all are equally important.

Policy-level action

As Bronfenbrenner (1979) pointed out (see Chapter 3), children's early experiences are shaped not simply by the *microsystems* and *mesosystem* around them, but also by the distant, invisible locations where blueprints for practice are laid down – the *macrosystem* of society as a whole and the *exosystem* where more local decisions are made. In early childhood provision, new policy initiatives have tumbled down to settings over the last few years, while local authorities and providers have had the task of interpreting them. Many governments, as we noticed in Chapter 4, are now listening to early years' practitioners, and responding positively to research evidence on the benefits for children of a more gradual induction into formal learning. In many countries, efforts are being made to carry the principles of early learning into elementary and primary schools, and to introduce children more slowly but more explicitly into formal learning styles and a subject-based curriculum.

This development is due in part to the recent emergence of strong leaders in the early years' field – advocates and researchers who are listened to by policy makers – an encouraging development in a domain which has traditionally tended to shy away from leadership (Mujis 2004; Rodd 2005). Changes in attitudes to children and families, and a more 'listening' culture, have been achieved by early years' practitioners and leaders speaking out, as individuals and through their professional organizations, and it is essential that we view such 'boldness' as part of our role. National policies, including new initiatives on funding, training and regulation, shape the provision offered to children and the frequency of their transitions; they also shape the experiences of providers and practitioners, who are themselves struggling to cope with constant change and short-lived initiatives. So this is an important area for continued action and pressure (including through research).

Provider-level action

School districts, municipalities and local authorities have also been persuaded by their practitioners of the need to take initiatives in mediating transitions, as the examples in Chapter 4 showed. Schools and settings can act alone, but funding for additional support and for research and publications are crucial in disseminating good practice such as that developed in Norfolk, Oxfordshire and Northern Ireland. In England, where government regulators inspect private, voluntary and independent settings, and local authorities are responsible for maintaining the quality of every kind of provision, opportunities exist for local advisers and pedagogues to raise the awareness of practitioners throughout the sector. Just as at the national level, strong and confident local leadership is required to ensure that young children and their families have a voice in decision making, and *all* practitioners need to see themselves as advocates (see Baldock et al. 2005).

School- and setting-level action

Individual schools and settings can do a great deal, through their own transition arrangements, to modify the shock of transitions between phases, whether from home to nursery, from nursery to school or within the school system. As we have seen, the earliest transitions are normally made with care and sensitivity, while later transitions may be viewed as more routine.

In England, as a result of concerns over the move into the formal phase of the National Curriculum, schools were offered training (*Continuing the Learning Journey*; QCA 2005) which encouraged them both to familiarize children with the phase to come, and to transfer many of their familiar experiences into the new classroom. Some schools devised a common, 'bridging' pedagogy which is introduced to children during their last two months in one phase (when their familiarity with their current environment and relationships supports their adaptation) and continues for the first two months in the subsequent phase (at which point they are acclimatized and ready for further innovations). Research in a sample of 12 schools (White and Sharp 2007) indicates some positive outcomes from such strategies. Many of the children interviewed identified quite small and unimportant differences when asked the question, *What's different about this year compared to last year?*

[Girl]   We *can* play in Year 1, but not lots of times any more.
[Boy]   Well, we have drawers now not a box for your book bag ...

On the whole, these organizational changes are acceptable because those interviewed understand the need for change, 'because you are getting older and growing up' (White and Sharp 2007: 87). Children in this study reported confidently on other transitional arrangements:

[Researcher] *What do you think it will be like in Year 1?*
[Girl] I already know because I have been there because we had 'change-over classes'.
[Boy] We went in their class already. Everybody moved up and I went in the Year 1 class.

Changes at this level are easily made, once children's concerns have been identified, and parents in the study confirmed the difference such practices had made to their children's understanding of what was expected of them.

Practitioner-level action

Practitioners' work with parents and with children is key to ensuring that positive and informative messages are conveyed from school to home, and that children and parents are listened to, throughout the transition process.

When children move from one phase to another, all the adults who are caring for them prepare them, consciously or unconsciously, for the unfamiliar environment that lies ahead; if the messages from 'home' and 'school' are similar, the changes may be more comprehensible and more acceptable. But as Gill Roberts (2007) reports, parents' perceptions are coloured by their vivid memories of fear and anxiety when they started school: 'The reasons for this, it seems, stemmed from not knowing what they should do, who they would be with or what would be expected of them'. These memories were rekindled when they saw their children facing the same challenge. As one parent reported, 'Teachers have that power. No matter how old you are, it's a throwback. You still feel it to some degree' (2007: 70). Most parents in this study had responded by discussing the changes to come with their child, and reminding them that these were the consequence of 'being big', but some had avoided mentioning it for fear of worrying the child in advance (2007: 72).

Practitioners need to recognize parents' own need for reassurance, and support their efforts to support their children: by treating parents with warmth and respect; explaining the changes to come very explicitly; and confirming that their child will continue to be valued as an individual. If children receive consistent explanations and information from the adults they trust, they can take their next steps with confidence.

Structural and cultural issues

It is important to remember that, despite the best efforts of policy makers, providers, practitioners, and parents, children do not enjoy equal opportunities to learn and succeed in their schools and pre-schools. Socioeconomic factors continue to have a strong association with children's academic progress and outcomes. They are evident when children start nursery (Sylva et al. 2004) and in their early school assessments: a study in Scotland reported that on entry to school, 'there were highly significant differences between the average scores of pupils from the groups with and without free school meals' (Tymms et al. 2005: 19). Poverty combines with other cultural factors to set obstacles in the path of some children. Transitions into settings which include more advantaged children may offer children new opportunities to flourish, or renewed experiences of exclusion. It would be wrong, however, to anticipate difficulties for all children from poor families: the story of Jelika (in Chapter 1) shows that children's own resources and resilience can overturn disadvantage. And so we turn to the other strand of this approach to transitions.

Strategies for 'positive outcomes': (ii) bestowing gifts and talents

It is technically quite incorrect to view adults as 'bestowing' characteristics on children, who are after all the main contributors to their own development and learning. Nevertheless, in thinking of what we 'want' for children, I find myself thinking of the gifts bestowed by the good and bad fairies on the infant Sleeping Beauty. We may lack magical powers, but we must use our own skills and talents to help children to develop theirs, and it is clear enough by now what these need to be. The 'gifts and talents' children require are those available to all children, and not just a select few (as Louis's nursery teachers recognized, in Chapter 4). We have identified resilience, resourcefulness and reciprocity; we could add, in support of strong children, two more essential Rs, and highlight the importance of reflection, and of rights.

Resilience

Resilience shows itself in many ways and is always impressive when we meet it in young or vulnerable children like Jelika. Its most accepted definition is that of Fonagy et al. (1994: 233): 'normal development under difficult circumstances', and Krovetz (1999) has identified four strands to this attribute: social competence, problem-solving skills, autonomy and a sense of purpose.

It is unlikely that all children can develop all these qualities at the same time or at the same pace; our role as adults is to be alert to any child's 'difficult circumstances' and to see which aspects of their resilience we can support and strengthen. For children like Jelika, access to familiar adults (family members) or to someone who spoke her language and could mediate the shock of school (bilingual support) would have made the transition less painful than it was, but the resources she summoned up from elsewhere enabled her to cope unaided. For many children, a secure environment and a sense of belonging are sufficient to enable them to work at difficulties. Here is Davey in his fourth week in Toddlers', displaying all of Krovetz's categories:

> He is pushing a very heavy wooden cart, making a real effort to push, then stop and redirect the steering, then move forward again. He looks in to check the contents: two paint brushes; moves forward a bit further then removes the brushes from the truck and walks purposefully to the back of the garden to the shed, which he then 'paints' with the brushes. Turns round, beaming with confidence and self-importance, and addresses other children to tell them what he is doing, pointing to the shed wall. Moves away a few feet to 'paint' the low posts round the sand pit, and then walks away to the slide.
>
> Stands at bottom of slide and 'paints' with brushes, using a damp patch on the slide surface to pick up a bit of moisture and spread it. 'Cleans' the brushes carefully with his fingers. Runs to the ladder on the slide and goes up carefully with a brush in each hand, so he can't hold on to the rails; gets on to the small platform at the top, sits there and then leans down to 'paint' the top part of the slide with his damp brush.
>
> Decides to go back down the ladder but has even more difficulty getting on to the ladder and down it with a brush in each hand (uses his elbows to wedge himself against the rails). Returns to the ground, walks round and 'paints' the slide again from the bottom end; stops, to allow a girl to slide down; then starts again.

Davey's key worker watched him from a distance but knew better than to intervene and 'help', or to engage him in conversation while he was involved. In this environment, Davey had the time, space and opportunities to use and strengthen his developing abilities, and his sense of achievement was evident.

Resourcefulness

Resourcefulness is another complex concept. As we saw in Chapter 3, it needs to be understood not simply as a quality 'in the child' but as a measure of the resources children can access in their environment. Piotrkowski's (2000) account of the way that poor families intuitively reckon the resources available to their own children – in the family, in the local childcare and education facilities, and in the neighbourhood more generally – makes good sense when we think of the different levels of 'resource' children have enjoyed before starting in school or pre-school. So educators need to attend to both kinds of resource: those available in the environment, ranging from blocks and paints to computers and adults, and those developing within the child, such as skills in problem solving and a disposition to work collaboratively. They need to be aware too that many of the resources children have acquired at home are derived from the family *habitus*, and are culturally appropriate within the child's community, but may not suit the culture of the school or setting.

Good-quality pre-school settings offer children both inner and outward resources. If we look again at Davey's story, we can see that his resources include:

- Access to time, space and a rich outdoor environment.
- Access to watchful and skilled practitioners.
- Opportunities to be involved alone or to interact with a peer group.
- Opportunities for problem solving within safe and secure boundaries.
- Opportunities to exercise his imagination with real-world materials.
- Opportunities for self-assessment and a sense of achievement.

This purposeful activity is described by sociocultural researchers in terms of the child's participation in a 'community of practice'. Davey undertakes his activity independently, but in doing so he is participating fully in the life of the small community which constitutes his world in the nursery; he knows that other children and adults are there to share in his efforts and celebrate his success. This experience is a rich resource which children like Davey will carry with them through their transitions into new learning environments, but the challenge for educators is to ensure that these new phases of learning offer children some of the same resources they have been used to – including adults they know they can turn to.

Reciprocity

This term sums up many of the skills that early educators and parents prioritize for children, and that will support children throughout their adult lives: sociability, perspective-taking, sharing, turn-taking, empathy and collaboration. Though these qualities develop 'within' the child they are acquired socially, and are nurtured and strengthened by involvement with peers.

The arrangements made by adults for the children in their care may leave such qualities to chance – and view some children as more or less sociable and cooperative than others – or they may be designed deliberately to provide opportunities for all children to develop reciprocity. As we have seen, even the youngest children seek friendly interactions with their peers, but practitioners may need to help some of them to be more aware of others. Here is Yuk-Yue in the first week of nursery:

> She and Shabna are sitting with Kerry, who is encouraging them to take pictures of each other with a digital camera. Yuk-Yue does not seem to be very interested in looking through the viewfinder and returns to busy herself organising plastic food on plastic plates. Kerry calls her back to see the picture Shabna has taken of her; she looks briefly before returning to the food

Kerry's observations of Yuk-Yue prompted her, a few weeks later, to undertake the series of cooking activities which helped all the children in her key group to become more aware of each other and of the experience of shared activity. As she explained, Yuk-Yue 'sometimes didn't have that time to bond with everyone ... so the cooking activity, they were sitting together, and they needed to pass things to one another, and that brought her in with the group'.

Experiencing the value of collaboration, and the pleasure of shared activity, is an early lesson which helps to form reciprocity in children. It is all the more important, then, that opportunities for group activities and shared efforts are not lost in subsequent phases, as learning becomes more individualized, and the learning environment competitive rather than collaborative.

Reflection

We are conscious of the need for practitioners to be 'reflective', but may not always prioritize this quality in children. Early induction into self-assessment practices – through a High/Scope style 'review' of achievements, a discussion for the portfolio, or a child conference designed to enhance metacognition – helps children acquire the habit of reflecting on *how* they have learned, as well as *what* they have learned. Children in the Valley School were confident in describing the mechanics of learning, even if their theorizing sounds unsophisticated in the light of adult knowledge: they were asked, 'How do you learn things?'

> *If you look at the shape, your brain tells you: it whispers in your ear and you think of doing it. Teachers and grown-ups tell you what to do, but you don't need teachers to teach you.*
>
> *(Sophie, 4 years 9 months)*
>
> *Some of my brain comes down from my head in my foot.*
>
> *(Joe, 5 years)*
>
> *You've got two brains and one squashy one which makes your brain go to sleep every night ... I been practising and practising and practising!*
>
> *(Cassie, 4 years 8 months)*

Children's misconceptions about learning (if indeed they *are* misconceptions) are unimportant: what matters is the act of thinking about thinking, and learning about learning. As children make successive transitions into new learning environments they need to carry with them a confident grasp of their own learning strategies – listening, thinking, copying, modelling, asking an adult, looking for a book, checking on the computer – as well as a sense of mastery about meeting new challenges.

Rights

As Chapter 5 argued, children's rights include participation rights, but in order to participate children must be informed of the relevant facts and circumstances, and helped to express their views in the best way they can.

Transition is an important time for the exercise of rights: children have the right to know, before they move to an unfamiliar environment, what this process will entail; the right to ask questions and seek explanations about the arrangements adults have made for them; and the right to express their views about these arrangements. 'Listening to children', it is clear, should be more than a token activity, and ideally should mean 'making common cause with children' – acting as advocates for their rights. Children's voices tell us much of what we need to know about making transitions work for them, and about sustaining their confidence and competence as learners in their new 'pupil' identities. The gradual loss of rights that children have described as they move through the school system is only gradually being addressed, but there is evidence that a culture of listening, and a belief that children have a valuable contribution to make, is spreading upwards through the system.

Working together for well-being

So far I have outlined the possibility of action at every level to alleviate some of the more serious discontinuities young children experience, and the indications that recent policy initiatives, nationally and inter-nationally, may contribute to this task. But in the end it is the 'team around the child', as *Every Child Matters* terms it, who will make the most difference for individual children, and the child's immediate care givers who are in the strongest position to act in his or her interests.

I conclude by looking again at these 'special people' and at the rela-tionships between them. Transitions have been described by Pianta et al. (1999: 72) as 'a process of relationship formation': 'the entry to Kinder-garten is fundamentally a matter of establishing a relationship between the home and the school in which the child's development is the key focus or goal'. But in consequence of differences in perspective, and cultural practices, such relationships are easily forged in some circum-stances, and fraught with difficulties in others. As Pianta et al. continue (1999: 72), the relationships are most important 'in cases in which social and economic resources are distributed differently between school and home, or are low', but this is precisely where they may be most difficult to construct and sustain.

Parents

Parents are the unsung heroes of young children's transitions: with few exceptions, and despite some anxieties and fears of their own, they work hard to prepare children for the changes in their lives. The ten 'case study' children described in this book all had parents who planned ahead conscientiously for the next stage of their child's development, according to their own beliefs about the child's best interests: they talked to them (or made them listen), encouraged them (or warned them), played with them (or made them 'study'), and instructed them in how to behave. When it came to making relationships with the staff of the school or setting, all of them did their best, and all of them expressed great trust and admiration for the key workers and teachers who looked after their children. But some – like Joshua's mother, and Saskia's – enjoyed instant rapport with the staff while others were inhibited by their own status or skills – like Jelika's mother, and Sonia's. Unless practitioners are given the time and space (and the leadership in their setting or school) to prioritize the task of establishing relationships with families who do not generally feel trusted and respected, the potential disadvantage to their children will accumulate through transitions into subsequent phases.

Key people

Recent policy developments have fostered a renewed emphasis on the 'key person' in each individual child's life. The Early Years Foundation Stage (*Practice Guidance*; DfES 2007: 19) defines such a person as the adult who 'shows a special interest in the child through close personal inter-action day-to-day' and also as 'the key point of contact with that child's parents' (*Statutory Framework*; DfES 2007: 52). The guidance emphasizes *secure attachment*, for school-age children as well as infants, *shared care* which supports the parent–child relationship, and the *independence* which the key-person relationship permits. Chapter 2 described a nursery – City Fields – which has already devoted thought and care to developing a key worker policy, and to ensuring that it is understood by all staff and parents, and applied throughout the centre.

Researchers with under-3s (Elfer et al. 2003) have shown how transitions within the setting can be managed in extended-day care, where staff working shifts cannot offer continuous care for a child, but a key person can be twinned with a 'buddy' who shares the care. Selleck (2006) contrasts this ideal – which the children's centres are intended to provide – with the 'serial care' offered in poor-quality settings, in which a child is handed on from one adult to another in the course of the day, or the week, or the month. Selleck advocates that pre-school settings are 'planned and managed so that each child experiences only a very few transitions of key person in the early years before entering a Key Stage 1 class – and none at all in one day at a setting' (2006: 12). Secure attachment to a key person, she suggests, may protect children from the damaging levels of stress-induced cortisone which are found in children, even in high-quality settings. But it can offer similar support to children who are outwardly more robust: school systems in which children 'change teacher' every year confront some children with anxiety and sometimes unhappiness on an annual basis, with a demonstrable impact on their progress (see Pollard and Filer 1999). Countries such as Denmark, where children stay with their educator for several years, affirm that the benefits outweigh any potential disadvantages but continuity for a shorter period can be arranged within existing systems through 'looping' arrangements in which teachers 'move up' with their children for one or two years. As with most of these options, a firm commitment and leadership in the school or setting is the key to overcoming barriers in the way of continuity.

Children

The 'triangle of care' discussed in Chapter 2 is associated with very young children, but we can envisage it as persisting, under various guises, throughout a child's school education. Lady Plowden (CACE 1967) used the idea of a triangle to argue for a close parent–teacher relationship, so that the flow of information and energy from parent to child, and from teacher to child, could be linked up like an electric circuit and thereby function more effectively. Children's own contribution to this relationship must not be ignored: from an early age they show themselves to be both capable and caring – for their care givers and for their peers. We do them an injustice if we construct them as weak, or as victims of their own circumstances, when – as Chapter 5 shows – they can speak out so effectively on their own behalf. As Dunlop and Fabian have said,

> The resilience, versatility and promise of young children as evidenced in their capacity to adapt to, to tolerate and especially to contribute to the creation and co-construction of the systems in which they live, grow and learn is central to any enquiry about educational transition.
>
> (2002: 131).

Conclusion

The 'recommendations' in this book may appear somewhat scattered, but as any reader will understand, they are summed up in the 'goals' for good transitions which this chapter has revisited. Practitioners and teachers are expert at working with individual children and key groups, and within their own room or school or setting, and do not need me to advise them on the day-to-day welcome they offer to children and families. But early years' educators do sometimes need to be reminded to raise their eyes and look over the fence: to take on responsibilities outside their classroom or setting; to challenge popular assumptions about young children's competence and their rights; to speak up in local associations and even advocate for support for children at a national level. Education is political, in the fullest sense of the word and at every level: it is about the power that is held by different individuals – adults and children, parents and practitioners – in relationship to each other.

Some of this power resides in words, and the meanings we give them: as Skinner et al. (1998: 308) affirm, 'ideas like "competence", "readiness", "risk" and "promise" are not entities located in the child but are cultural and historical constructions produced in everyday practices and within larger systems'. The case studies in this book have tried to demonstrate this fact: that the knowledge, skills and dispositions children possess are always viewed through the lens of our own national and local 'arrangements' for children. These arrangements in the end derive from public policy for children, and we should all do our best to influence that.

> In framing the transition issue for the public and the media, early childhood leaders should emphasize the long-term benefits for children and parents of investing in transition activities ... the public needs to know that investment in transitions is cost-effective. Activities to promote successful transitions are often inexpensive, yet they are critical to maximizing the development of young children.
>
> (Kagan and Neuman 1998: 373)

The message is clear: in supporting transitions, we all need to be early childhood leaders.

References

Ainsworth, M. (1978) *Patterns of Attachment*. Mahwah, NJ: Lawrence Erlbaum Associates.

Alderson, P. (2000) *Young Children's Rights*. London: Jessica Kingsley.

Alderson, P. (2002) Students' rights in British schools: trust, autonomy, connection and regulation, in R. Edwards (ed.) *Children, Home and School*. London: RoutledgeFalmer.

Alderson, P., Hawthorne, J. and Killen, M. (2005) The participation rights of premature babies, *International Journal of Children's Rights*, 13: 31–50.

Ames, C. (1992) Classrooms: goals, structures and student motivation, *Journal of Educational Psychology*, 84(3): 261–71.

Anning, A. (1991) *The First Years at School*. Milton Keynes: Open University Press.

Arnold, C., Bartlett, K., Gowani, S. and Merali, R. (2006) *Is Everybody Ready? Readiness, Transition and Continuity: Lessons, Reflections and Moving Forward*. Paper commissioned for the EFA Global Monitoring report 2007, Strong Foundations: Early Childhood Care and Education.

Baldock, P., Fitzgerald, D. and Kay, J. (2005) *Understanding Early Years Policy*. London: Paul Chapman.

Barrett, G. (1986) *Starting School: An Evaluation of the Experience*. London: AMMA.

Barrett, G. (ed.) (1989) *Disaffection from School? The Early Years*. London: Falmer.

Bennett, J. (2006) An interview with John Bennett, *Early Childhood Matters*, 107: 13–19.

Bennett, N. and Kell, J. (1989) *A Good Start? Four Year Olds in Infant School*. Oxford: Blackwell.

Bennett, N., Wood, L. and Rogers, S. (1997) *Teaching Through Play*. Buckingham: Open University Press.

Bernstein, B. (1970) Education cannot compensate for society, *New Society*, 26 February.

Bernstein, B. (1971) *Class, Codes and Control: Theoretical Studies Towards a Sociology of Language*. London: Routledge and Kegan Paul.

Bernstein, B. (1975) *Class, Codes and Control: Towards a Theory of Educational Transmissions*. London: Routledge and Kegan Paul.

Bertram, T. and Pascal, C. (2002) *Early Years Education: An International Perspective*. London: QCA.

Black, P. and Wiliam, D. (1998) Assessment and classroom learning, *Assessment in Education*, 5(1): 7–44.

Black, O., Harrison, C., Lee, C. et al. (2004) Working inside the black box: assessment for learning in the classroom, *Phi Delta Kappan*, 86.

Blatchford, P., Battle, S. and Mays, J (1982) *The First Transition: Home to Preschool*. Windsor: NFER-Nelson.

Bourdieu, P. (1986) The forms of capital, in A. Halsey, H. Lauder, P. Brown and A. Wells (eds) *Education, Culture, Economy, Society*. Oxford: Oxford University Press.

Bourdieu, P. (1990a) *The Logic of Practice*. Cambridge: Polity.

Bourdieu, P. (1990b) *In Other Words: Essays Towards a Reflexive Sociology*. Cambridge: Polity.

Bourdieu, P. and Wacquant, L. (1992) *Invitation to Reflexive Sociology*. Bristol: Policy Press.

Bowlby, J. (1978) *Separation: Anxiety and Anger*. Harmondsworth: Penguin.

Brannen, J. and Moss, P. (eds) (2003) *Rethinking Children's Care*. Buckingham: Open University Press.

Bronfenbrenner, U. (1979) *The Ecology of Human Development*. Cambridge, MA: Harvard University Press.

Brooker, L. (1996) Why do children go to school? Consulting children in the reception class, *Early Years*, 17(1): 12–16.

Brooker, L. (2001) Interviewing children, in G. MacNaughton, S. Rolfe and I. Siraj-Blatchford (eds) *Doing Early Childhood Research*. Sydney: Allen and Unwin.

Brooker, L. (2002) *Starting School: Young Children Learning Cultures*. Buckingham: Open University Press.

Brooker, L. (2006) From home to the home corner: observing children's identity-maintenance in early childhood settings, *Children and Society*, 20: 116–27.

Brooker, L. and Broadbent, L. (2007) Personal, social and emotional development: learning to be strong in a world of change, in J. Riley (ed.) *Learning in the Early Years*. London: Sage.

Broström, S. (2002) Communication and continuity in the transition from kindergarten to school, in H. Fabian and A.-W. Dunlop (eds) *Transitions in the Early Years*. London: RoutledgeFalmer.

Bruer, J. (1999) Neural connections: some you use, some you lose, *Phi Delta Kappan*, 81(4): 264–77.

Bruner, J. (1996) *The Culture of Education*. Cambridge, MA: Harvard University Press.

Buchbinder, M., Longhofer, J., Barrett, T., Lawson, P. and Floersch, J. (2006) Ethnographic approaches to child care research: a review of the literature, *Journal of Early Childhood Research*, 4(1): 45–63.

Burrell, A. and Bubb, S. (2000) Teacher feedback in the reception class: associations with children's positive adjustment to school, *Education 3–13*, (October): 58–64.

Carmichael, E. and Hancock, J. (2007) Scotland, in M. Clark and T. Waller (eds) *Early Childhood Education and Care*. London: Sage.

Carr, M. (2001) *Assessment in Early Childhood Settings*. London: Paul Chapman.

Carr, M., Jones, C. and Lee, W. (2005) Beyond listening: can assessment practice play a part?, in A. Clark, A.-T. Kjørholt and P. Moss (eds) *Beyond Listening: Children's Perspectives on Early Childhood Services*. Bristol: Policy Press.

Central Advisory Committee for Education (CACE) (1967) *Children and Their Primary Schools*. London: HMSO.

Clark, A. (2005) Ways of seeing: using the MOSAIC approach to listen to young children's perspectives, in A. Clark, A.-T. Kjørholt and P. Moss (eds) *Beyond Listening: Children's Perspectives on Early Childhood Services*. Bristol: Policy Press.

Clark, A. and Moss, P. (2001) *Listening to Children: The MOSAIC Approach*. London: National Children's Bureau.

Claxton, G. (1995) What kind of learning does self-assessment drive? *Assessment in Education*, 2(3): 339–43.

Cleave, S., Jowett, S. and Bate, M. (1982) *And So to School: A Study of Continuity from Pre-school to Infant School*. Berkshire: NFER-Nelson.

Cole, M. (1998) Culture in development, in M. Woodhead, D. Faulkner and K. Littleton (eds) *Cultural Worlds of Early Childhood*. London: Routledge/Open University Press.

Committee on the Rights of the Child (CRC) (2005) *General Comment 7: Implementing Child Rights in Early Childhood*. Geneva: United Nations.

Corsaro, W., Molinari, L., Hadley, K. and Sugioka, H. (2003) Keeping and making friends: Italian children's transition from preschool to elementary school, *Social Psychology Quarterly*, 66(3): 272–91.

Cowie, B. and Carr, M. (2004) The consequences of sociocultural assessment, in A. Anning, J. Cullen and M. Fleer (eds) *Early Childhood Education: Society and Culture*. London: Sage.

Dalli, C. (1999) Learning to be in childcare: mothers' stories of their child's settling-in, *European Early Childhood Education Research Journal*, 7(2), 53–66.

Dalli, C. (2000) Starting child care: what young children learn about relating to adults in the first weeks of starting child care, *Early Childhood Research and Practice*, 2(2): 1–31.

Daniel, J. (1998) A modern mother's place is wherever her children are: facilitating infant and toddler mothers' transitions in child care, *Young Children*, Nov: 4–12.

Daniel, J. and Shapiro, J. (1996) Infant transitions: home to centre-based child care, *Child and Youth Care Forum*, 25(2): 111–23.

Department for Education and Skills (2002) *Birth to Three Matters: A Framework to Support Children in Their Earliest Years*, London: DfES/Sure Start Unit.

Department for Education and Skills (DfES) (2003a) *Foundation Stage Profile Handbook*. London: QCA.

Department for Education and Skills (DfES) (2003b) *Every Child Matters*. Norwich: The Stationery Office.

Department for Education and Skills (2007) *Early Years Foundation Stage (Practice Guidance)*. Nottingham: DfES Publications.

Department for Education and Skills/Qualifications and Curriculum Authority (DfES/QCA) (2000) *Curriculum Guidance for the Foundation Stage*. London: DfES.

Dockett, S. and Perry, B. (2002) Who's ready for what? Young children starting school, *Contemporary Issues in Early Childhood*, 3(1): 67–89.

Dockett, S. and Perry, B. (2004) What makes a successful transition to school? Views of Australian parents and teachers, *International Journal of Early Years Education*, 12(3): 217–30.

Dockett, S. and Perry, B. (2005a) Starting school in Australia is 'a bit safer, a lot easier and more relaxing': issues for families and children from culturally and linguistically diverse backgrounds, *Early Years*, 25(3): 271–81.

Dockett, S. and Perry, B. (2005b) 'You need to know how to play safe': children's experiences of starting school, *Contemporary Issues in Early Childhood*, 6(1): 4–18.

Dockett, S. and Perry, B. (2007) Children's transition to school: changing expectations, in A.-W. Dunlop and H. Fabian (eds) *Informing Transitions in the Early Years*. Maidenhead: Open University Press.

Dockett, S., Perry, B., Howard, P., Whitton, D. and Cusack, M. (2002) Australian children starting school, *Childhood Education: International Focus Issue*, 349–53.

Donaldson, M. (1978) *Children's Minds*. London: Flamingo.

Dowling, M. (1995) *Starting School at Four: A Joint Endeavour*. London: Paul Chapman.

Drummond, M. J. (2003) *Assessing Children's Learning*. London: David Fulton.

Dunn, J. (2004) *Children's Friendships: The Beginnings of Intimacy*. Oxford: Blackwell.

Dweck, C. and Leggett, E. (1988) A socio-cognitive approach to motivation and achievement, *Psychological Review*, 95(2): 256–73.

Elfer, P., Goldschmied, E. and Selleck, D. (2003) *Key Persons in the Nursery: Building Relationships for Quality Provision*. London: David Fulton.

Eide, B. and Winger, N. (2005) From the children's point of view: methodological and ethical challenges, in A. Clark, A.-T. Kjørholt and P. Moss (eds) *Beyond Listening: Children's Perspectives on Early Childhood Services*. Bristol: Policy Press.

Einarsdottir, J. (2007) Children's voices on the transition from preschool to primary school, in A.-W. Dunlop and H. Fabian (eds) *Informing Transitions in the Early Years*. Maidenhead: McGraw-Hill.

Entwisle, D. and Alexander, K. (1998) Facilitating the transition to first grade: the nature of transition and research on factors affecting it, *Elementary School Journal*, 98(4): 351–64.

Eyre, D. (1997) *Able Children in Ordinary Schools*. London: David Fulton.

Fabian, H. (1996) Children starting school: parents in partnership, *Mentoring and Tutoring*, 4(1): 12–22.

Fabian, H. and Dunlop, A.-W. (eds) (2002) *Transitions in the Early Years*. London: RoutledgeFalmer.

Fabian, H. and Dunlop, A.-W. (2006) *Outcomes of Good Practice in Transition Processes for Children Entering Primary School*. Paper commissioned for the EFA Global Monitoring Report, 2007, *Strong Foundations: Early Childhood Care and Education*.

Faulkner, D. and Miell, D. (1993) Settling into school: the importance of early friendships, *International Journal of Early Years Education*, 1(1): 23–45.

Fisher. J. (2006) Handle with care! Transitions in the early years, *Early Education*, Autumn: 7–10.

Fleer, M. (2002) Sociocultural assessment in early years education: myth or reality? *International Journal of Early Years Education*, 10(2): 105–20.

Fleer, M. and Richardson, C. (2004) Mapping the transformation of understanding, in A. Anning, J. Cullen and M. Fleer (eds) *Early Childhood Education: Society and Culture*. London: Sage.

Fonagy, P., Steele, M., Steele, H., Higgit, A. and Target, M. (1994) The theory and practice of resilience, *Journal of Child Psychology and Psychiatry*, 35(2): 231–57.

Fthenakis, W. (1998) Family transitions and quality in early childhood education, *European Early Childhood Education Research Journal*, 6(1): 5–17.

Gagne, F. (1991) Toward a differentiated model of giftedness and talent, in N. Colangela and G. Davis (eds) *Handbook of Gifted Education*. Boston, MA: Allyn and Bacon.

Ghuman, P. and Gallop, R. (1981) Educational attitudes of Bengali families in Cardiff, *Journal of Multicultural and Multilingual Development*, 2(2): 127–44.

Ghuman, P. and Wong, R. (1989) Chinese parents and English education, *Educational Research*, 31(2): 134–40.

Gill, S., Winters, D. and Friedman, D. (2006) Educators' views of pre-kindergarten and kindergarten readiness and transition practices, *Contemporary Issues in Early Childhood*, 7(3): 213–27.

Gipps, C. (2002) Sociocultural perspectives on assessment, in G. Wells and G. Claxton (eds) *Learning for Life in the 21st Century*. Oxford: Blackwell.

Goldschmied, E. and Jackson, S. (2004) *People Under Three: Young Children in Day Care*. London: Routledge.

Green, D. and Lepper, M. (1974) How to turn play into work, *Psychology Today*, 8(4): 49–54.

Gregory, E. and Biarnes, J. (1994) Tony and Jean Francois looking for sense in the strangeness of school, in H. Dombey and M. Spenser (eds) *First Steps Together*. Stoke-on-Trent: Trentham Books.

Gura, P. (1996) What I want for Cinderella: self-esteem and self-assessment, *Early Education*, 19: 3–5.

Harkness, S. (1980) The cultural context of child development, *New Directions for Child Development*, 8: 7–13.

Heath, S.B. (1983) *Ways with Words: Language, Life and Work in Communities and Classroom*. Cambridge: Cambridge University Press.

Hendy, L. and Whitebread, D. (2000) Interpretations of independent learning in the early years, *International Journal of Early Years Education*, 8(3): 243–52.

Hitz, R. and Driscoll, A. (1988) Praise or encouragement? *Young Children*, July: 6–13.

Hohmann, U. (2007) Rights, expertise and negotiations in care and education, *Early Years*, 27(1): 33–46.

Hubbell, R., Plantz, R., Cobdelli, L. and Barrett, B. (1987) *The transition of Head Start children into public school*, Final report. Alexandria, VA: CSR.

Hughes, M., Pinkerton, G. and Plewis, I. (1979) Children's difficulties on starting infant school, *Journal of Child Psychology and Psychiatry*, 20: 187–96.

Jackson, B. (1979) *Starting School*. London: Croom Helm.

Jackson, C. and Warin, J. (2000) The importance of gender as an aspect of identity at key transition points in compulsory education, *British Educational Research Journal*, 26(3): 375–91.

Kagan, S. and Neuman, M. (1998) Lessons from three decades of transition research, *Elementary School Journal*, 98(4): 365–79.

Kagan, S. (1999) Cracking the readiness mystique, *Young Children*, (September): 2–3.

Kavkoulis, A. (1994) Continuity in early childhood education: transition from pre-school to school, *International Journal of Early Years Education*, 2(1): 41–51.

Katz, L. (1994) *Talks with Teachers of Young Children*. Norwood, NJ: Ablex.

Kitson, R. (2004) Starting school in Brunei: listening to children, parents and teachers, *Contemporary Issues in Early Childhood*, 5(2): 236–42.

Krovetz, M. (1999) *Fostering Resiliency*. California: Corwen Press.

Laevers, F. and Heylen, L. (eds) (2003) *Involvement of Children and Teacher Style: Insights from an International Study of Experiential Education*. Leuven: Leuven University Press.

Laming, Lord (2003) *The Victoria Climbie Inquiry Report*. Norwich: HMSO.

La Paro, L., Pianta, R. and Cox, M. (2000) Kindergarten teachers' reported use of kindergarten to first grade transition practices, *Elementary School Journal*, 101(1): 63–78.

Lave, J. and Wenger, E. (1991) *Situated Learning: Legitimate Peripheral Participation*. Cambridge: Cambridge University Press.

Love, J., Logue, M., Trudeau, J. and Thayer, K. (1992) *Transitions to Kindergarten in American Schools. Final Report of the National Transition Study*. Portsmouth, NH: RMC Research Corp.

Mangione, P. and Speth, T. (1998) The transition to elementary school: a framework for creating early childhood continuity through home, school and community partnerships, *Elementary School Journal*, 98(4): 381–97.

Mayall, B. (2002) *Towards a Sociology for Childhood: Thinking From Children's Lives*. Buckingham: Open University Press.

Michaels, S. (1986) Narrative presentations: an oral preparation for literacy with first graders, in J. Cook-Gumperz (ed.) *The Social Construction of Literacy.* Cambridge: Cambridge University Press.

Moss, P., Clark, A. and Kjørholt, A.-T. (2005) Introduction, in A. Clark, A.-T. Kjørholt and P. Moss (eds) *Beyond Listening: Children's Perspectives on Early Childhood Services.* Bristol: Policy Press.

Mujis, D., Aubrey, C., Harris, A. and Briggs, M. (2004) How do they manage? A review of the research on leadership in early childhood, *Journal of Early Childhood Research,* 2(2): 157–69.

Murray, L. and Andrews, L. (2000) *The Social Baby.* Richmond: CP Publishing.

Myers, R. (1992) *The Twelve Who Survive: Strengthening Programmes of Early Childhood Development in the Third World.* London: Routledge.

National Education Goals Panel (1991) *The National Education Goals Report.* Washington, DC: National Education Goals Panel.

Neuman, M. (2001) *Early Childhood Education: Critical Perspectives.* Paris: OECD.

Newson, E. and Newson, J. (1968) *Four Years Old in an Urban Community.* London: Allen and Unwin.

Newson, E. and Newson, J. (1976) *Seven Years Old in the Home Environment.* Harmondsworth: Penguin.

Niesel, R. and Griebel, W. (2005) Transitions competence and resiliency in educational institutions, *International Journal of Transitions in Childhood,* 1(1): 4–11.

New Zealand Ministry of Education (1996) *Te Whariki: Early Childhood Curriculum.* Wellington: Learning Media.

New Zealand Ministry of Education (2006) *The New Zealand Curriculum Draft for Consultation.* Wellington: Learning Media.

O'Kane, M. and Hayes, N. (2007) The transition to school in Ireland: what do the children say? Paper presented at the CECDE International Conference, 'Vision into Practice', Dublin, Ireland.

O'Kane, M. (2007) Children's interview data [personal communication].

Oxfordshire County Council (2006) *Transition, Foundation Stage to Year 1.* Oxford: Oxfordshire County Council.

Pascal, C. and Bertram, T. (1997) *Effective Early Learning: Case Studies in Improvement.* London: Hodder and Stoughton.

Peters, S. (2007) Responsive, reciprocal relationships: the heart of the *Te Whaariki* curriculum. Paper presented at the 'Reclaiming Relational Pedagogy' Conference, Chelmsford.

Petriwskyj, A., Thorpe, K. and Tayler, C. (2005) Trends in construction of transition to school in three western regions, *International Journal of Early Years Education,* 13(1): 55–69.

Pianta, R. and Cox, M. (eds) (1999) *The Transition to Kindergarten.* Baltimore, MD: Paul Brookes.

Pianta, R., Cox, M., Taylor, L., and Early, D. (1999) Kindergarten teachers' practices related to the transition to school: results of a national survey, *Elementary School Journal,* 100(1): 71–86.

Piotrkowski, C., Botsko, M. and Matthews, E. (2000) Parents' and teachers' beliefs about children's school readiness in a high-need community, *Early Childhood Research Quarterly*, 15(4): 537–58.

Pluckrose, H. (1987) *What Is Happening in Our Primary Schools?* Oxford: Basil Blackwell.

Pollard, A. and Filer, A. (1999) *The Social World of Pupil Career*. London: Cassell.

Pollard, A. with Filer, A. (1996) *The Social World of Children's Learning: Case Studies of Pupils from Four to Seven*. London: Cassell.

Pollard, A., Broadfoot, P., Croll, P., Osborn, M. and Abbott, D. (1994) *Changing English Primary Schools? The Impact of the Education Reform Act at Key Stage One*. London: Cassell.

Pugh, G. (2002) The consequences of a failure to invest in early learning, in J. Fisher (ed.) *The Foundations of Learning*. Buckingham: Open University Press.

Qualifications and Curriculum Authority (QCA) (2005) *Continuing the Learning Journey*. London: QCA

Quick, S., Lambley, C., Newcombe, E. and Aubrey, C. (2002) *Implementing the Foundation Stage in Reception Classes*. DfES Research Report 350. London: DfES.

Ramey, S. and Ramey, C. (1998) Commentary: the transition to school: opportunities and challenges for children, families, educators and communities, *Elementary School Journal*, 98(4): 293–5.

Ramey, S., Lanzi, R., Phillips, M., Ramey, C. (1998) Perspectives of former Head Start children and their parents on school and the transition to school, *Elementary School Journal*, 98(4): 311–27.

Rimm-Kaufman, S., Pianta, R. and Cox, M. (2000) Teachers' judgments of problems in the transition to kindergarten, *Early Childhood Research Quarterly*, 15(2): 147–66.

Rinaldi, C. (2005) Documentation and assessment: what is the relationship? in A. Clark, A.-T. Kjørholt and P. Moss (eds) *Beyond Listening: Children's Perspectives on Preschool Services*. Bristol: Policy Press.

Rist, R. (1970) Student social class and teacher expectation: the self-fulfilling prophecy in ghetto education, *Harvard Educational Review*, 40(3): 411–51.

Roberts, G. (2007) *Transition from the Foundation Stage into Key Stage 1*, University of London, Institute of Education, unpublished MA dissertation.

Roberts, R. (2002) *Self-esteem and Early Learning*. London: Paul Chapman Publishing.

Rodd, J. (2005) *Leadership in Early Childhood*. Buckingham: Open University Press.

Rogoff, B. (1990) *Apprenticeship in Thinking: Cognitive Development in Social Context*. Oxford: Oxford University Press.

Rogoff, B., Mistry, J., Göncü, A. and Mosier, C. (1993) Guided participation in cultural activity by toddlers and caregivers, *Monograph of the Society for Research and Child Development*, 58(7).

Rosenthal, R. and Jacobson, L. (1968) *Pygmalion in the Classroom: Teacher Expectation and Pupils' Intellectual Development*. New York: Holt, Rinehart, Winston.

Rutter, M. (2000) Resilience reconsidered: conceptual considerations, empirical findings, and policy implications, in J.P. Shonkoff and S.J. Meisels (eds)

Handbook of Early Childhood Intervention. Cambridge: Cambridge University Press.

Saluja, G., Scott-Little, C. and Clifford, M. (2000) Readiness for school: a survey of state policies and definitions, *Early Childhood Research and Practice*, 2(2): 1–15.

Schaffer, H.R. (1996) *Social Development.* Oxford: Blackwell.

Schieffelin, B. and Ochs, E. (1986) *Language Socialization Across Cultures.* New York: Cambridge University Press.

Schweinhart, L., Montie, J., Xiang, Z. et al. (2004) *Lifetime Effects: The High/Scope Perry Preschool Study Through Age 40.* Ypsilanti, MI: High/Scope Press.

Selleck, D. (2006) Key persons in the Early Years Foundation Stage, *Early Education*, 50 (Autumn): 11–13.

Sevenhuijsen, S. (1999) *Citizenship and the Ethics of Care.* London: Routledge.

Sharp, C. (2002) *School Starting Age: European Policy and Recent Research.* Paper presented at LGA Seminar, November 2002.

Shonkoff, J. and Phillips, D. (eds) (2000) *From Neurons to Neighbourhoods: The Science of Early Childhood Development.* Washington, DC: Board on Children, Youth and Families; Committee on Integrating the Science of Early Childhood Development.

Siraj-Blatchford, I., Sylva, K.,Laugharne, J., Milton, E. and Charles, F. (2006) *Monitoring and Evaluation of the Effective Implementation of the Foundation Phase Project Across Wales.* London: Institute of Education.

Skinner, D., Bryant, D., Coffman, J. and Campbell, F. (1998) Creating risk and promise: children's and teachers' co-constructions in the cultural world of kindergarten, *Elementary School Journal*, 98(4): 297–310.

Smiley, P. and Dweck, C. (1994) Individual differences in achievement goals among young children, *Child Development*, 65(6): 1723–43.

Super, C. and Harkness, S. (1977) The infant's niche in rural Kenya and metropolitan America, in L. Adler (ed.) *Issues in Cross-cultural Research.* New York: Academic Press.

Super, C. and Harkness, S. (1998) The development of affect in infancy and early childhood, in M. Woodhead, D. Faulkner and K. Littleton (eds) *Cultural Worlds of Early Childhood.* London: Routledge/Open University.

Sylva, K. (1994) The impact of early learning on children's later development, in C. Ball (ed.) *Start Right: The Importance of Early Learning.* London: Royal Society of Arts.

Sylva, K., Melhuish, E., Sammons, P., Siraj-Blatchford, I. and Taggart, B. (2004) *Final Report, Effective Provision of Preschool Education.* London: Institute of Education.

Thyssen, S. (2000) The child's start in day care centre; *Early Child Development and Care*, 161: 33–46.

Tizard, B. and Hughes, M. (1984) *Young Children Learning.* London: Fontana.

Tizard, B., Blatchford, P., et al. (1988) *Young Children at School in the Inner City.* London: Lawrence Erlbaum.

Torrance, H. and Pryor, J. (2004) Investigating formative classroom assessment, in

L. Polson and M. Wallace (eds) *Learning to Read Critically in Teaching and Learning*. London: Sage

Trevarthen, C. (1998) The child's need to learn a culture, in M. Woodhead, D. Faulkner and K. Littleton (eds) *Cultural Worlds of Early Childhood*. London: RoutledgeFalmer.

Tronto, J. (1993) *Moral Boundaries: A Political Argument for the Ethics of Care*. London: Routledge.

Tunstall, P. and Gipps, C. (1996) Teacher feedback to young children in formative assessment: a typology, *British Educational Research Journal*, 22(4): 389–404.

Tymms, P. and Merrell, C. (2004) On-entry baseline assessment across cultures, in A. Anning, J. Cullen and M.Fleer (eds) *Early Childhood Education: Society and Culture*. London: Sage.

Tymms, P., Jones, P., Merrell, C., Henderson, B. and Cowie, M. (2005) *Children Starting School in Scotland*. Edinburgh: Scottish Executive Education Department.

United Nations (1989) *Convention on the Rights of the Child*. Geneva: United Nations.

Vinovskis, M. (2005) *The Birth of Head Start*. Chicago: University of Chicago Press.

Vygotsky, L. (1978) *Mind in Society: The Development of Higher Psychological Processes*. Cambridge, MA: Harvard University Press.

Vygotsky, L. (1962) *Thought and Language*. Cambridge, MA: MIT Press.

Walsh, G. (2007) Northern Ireland, in M. Clark and T. Waller (eds) *Early Childhood Education and Care: Policy and Practice*. London: Sage.

Warming, H. (2005) Participant observation: a way to learn about children's perspectives, in A. Clark, A.-T. Kjørholt and P. Moss (eds) *Beyond Listening: Children's Perspectives on Early Childhood Services*. Bristol: Policy Press.

Waterhouse, S. (1991) *First Episodes: Pupil Careers in the Early Years of School*. London: Falmer.

Wells, G. (1985) *The Meaning Makers*. London: Hodder and Stoughton.

Wells, G. and Claxton, G. (2002) *Learning for Life in the Twenty-first Century*. Oxford: Blackwell.

Welsh Assembly Government (2003) *The Learning Country: The Foundation Phase – 3 to 7 years*. Cardiff: National Assembly for Wales.

Whalley, M. (2007) *Involving Parents in their Children's Learning*. London: Sage.

White, G. and Sharp, C. (2007) 'It is different . . . because you are getting older and growing up'. How children make sense of the transition to Year 1, *European Early Childhood Education Research Journal*, 15(1): 87–102.

Williams, R. (1976) *Key Words*. London: Fontana.

Wood, D. (1998) *How Children Think and Learn*. Oxford: Blackwell.

Woodhead, M. (1989) School starts at 5 . . . or 4 years old? The rationale for changing admission policy in England and Wales, *Journal of Education Policy*, 4: 1–22.

Woodhead, M. (1996) *In Search of the Rainbow*. The Hague: Bernard van Leer Foundation.

Index

EARLY YEARS FOUNDATIONS
Meeting the Challenge

Janet Moyles

Using the new *Early Years Foundation Stage* principles as its framework, the contributors support early years professionals in dealing with issues and challenges in a sensitive and professional manner, with particular emphasis upon the need for practitioners to personalise the requirements for each child in their care and to reflect closely upon their own and children's experiences.

Topics include: the changing landscape of early childhood, culture, identity and diversity, supporting playful learning, outdoor learning, documenting children's experiences, developing independence in learning, the meaning of being creative, play and mark-making in maths, and literacy.

Each section is introduced with some background research and information to provide evidence and guidance upon which practitioners can make their own decisions. Individual chapters include questions for reflection, points for discussion and suggestions for additional reading.

Early Years Foundations: Meeting the Challenge is essential reading for the full range of practitioners working and playing with birth-to-five-year-olds.

2007   308pp
978-0-335-22349-7 (Paperback)   978-0-335-22348-0 (Hardback)

INFORMING TRANSITIONS IN THE EARLY YEARS
Research, Policy and Practice

Aline-Wendy Dunlop and Hilary Fabian (eds)

This book explores early transitions from a variety of international perspectives. Each chapter is informed by rigorous research and makes recommendations on how education professionals can better understand and support transitions in the early years. Contributors examine issues such as:

- Parental involvement in the transition to school

- Children's voices on the transition to primary school

- The construction of identity in the early years

Readers will be able to draw support, guidance and inspiration from the different writers to scaffold their own thinking and development in relation to children's transitions. Ample opportunities are offered for readers to gain confidence and competence in dealing with the range of people involved in transitions, and to the benefit of everyone, not least the children, whose 'transitions capital' will grow.

Contents: *List of contributors - Preface - Foreword - Acknowledgements - Introduction - Informing Transitions - Models of Transition - Enhancing the competence of transition systems through co-construction - Horizontal transitions: What can it mean for children in the early school years? - The construction of different identities within an early childhood centre: A case study - Children Experiencing Transition - Transitions in children's thinking - Children's voices on the transition from preschool to primary school - Children's transition to school: Changing expectations - Parents and Professionals Supporting Transitions - Understanding and supporting children: Shaping transition practices - Parent involvement in the transition to school - Expectations: Effects of curriculum change as viewed by children, parents and practitioners - Conclusion - Bridging research, policy and practice - Index.*

2006   176pp
978-0-335-22013-7 (Paperback)   978-0-335-22014-4 (Hardback)

CHILD DEVELOPMENT FROM BIRTH TO EIGHT
A Journey through the Early Years

Maria Robinson

Understanding child development is crucial for all early years practitioners and a sound knowledge of children and their development underpins effective practice.

The book presents a detailed and in-depth picture of early years development, particularly of developmental processes and interactions. Rather than focusing on a particular topic, it offers a broad overview from a range of sources including:

- Developmental, evolutionary and cognitive psychology
- Biology
- Sensory information
- Attachment theory
- Neuroscience
- Research linking brain function and emotions

As well as providing a great insight into the aspects of child development and offering the benefits of a multi-disciplinary approach, the book emphasizes appropriate pedagogical approaches and the implications for adults who work with young children.

Child Development from Birth to Eight is essential reading for all early years students and practitioners.

Contents: *Foreword - Acknowledgements - Introduction - Laying the foundations: Brain works - 'A world of one's own': The body and the senses - Origins - Emotional and social and well being - Learning and development - Playing and imagining - The role of the adult: To understand the 'heart of the intended communication' - The final phase, conclusions and reflections on development - Appendix - Glossary - Notes - Bibliography - Index.*

2007   584pp
978-0-335-22097-7 (Paperback)   978-0-335-22098-4 (Hardback)

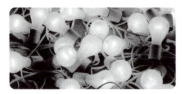
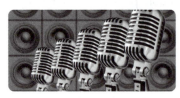
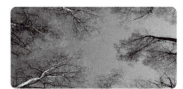
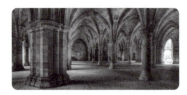
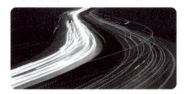
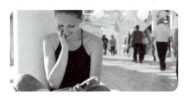
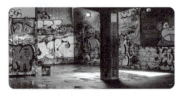
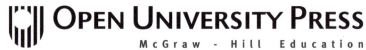